CW00498726

Supporting Staff Mental Health in Your School

of related interest

The Mentally Healthy Schools Workbook
Practical Tips, Ideas, Action Plans and Worksheets for Making Meaningful Change
Pooky Knightsmith
Foreword by Norman Lamb
ISBN 978 1 78775 148 4
eISBN 978 1 78775 149 1

The Mental Health and Wellbeing Handbook for Schools
Transforming Mental Health Support on a Budget
Clare Erasmus
Foreword by Chris Edwards
ISBN 978 1 78592 481 1
eISBN 978 1 78450 869 2

How to Be a Peaceful School
Practical Ideas, Stories and Inspiration
Edited by Anna Lubelska
ISBN 978 1 78592 156 8
eISBN 978 1 78450 424 3

Promoting Emotional Wellbeing in Early Years Staff
A Practical Guide for Looking After Yourself and Your Colleagues
Sonia Mainstone-Cotton
ISBN 978 1 78592 335 7
eISBN 978 1 78450 656 8

Mindful Co-Working
Be Confident, Happy and Productive in Your Working Relationships
Clark Baim
ISBN 978 1 84905 413 3
eISBN 978 0 85700 803 9

Supporting Staff Mental Health in Your School

Amy Sayer

Foreword by Pooky Knightsmith

Jessica Kingsley Publishers
London and Philadelphia

First published in Great Britain in 2021 by Jessica Kingsley Publishers
An Hachette Company

1

A CIP catalogue record for this title is available from the British Library and the Library of Congress

ISBN 978 1 78775 463 8
eISBN 978 1 78775 464 5

Printed and bound in Great Britain by Clays Ltd

Jessica Kingsley Publishers' policy is to use papers that are natural, renewable and recyclable products and made from wood grown in sustainable forests. The logging and manufacturing processes are expected to conform to the environmental regulations of the country of origin.

Jessica Kingsley Publishers
Carmelite House
50 Victoria Embankment
London EC4Y 0DZ

www.jkp.com

Contents

Foreword by Pooky Knightsmith 9

Preface 11

Introduction 17

Chapter 1 Common Types of Mental Ill Health among School Staff 31

Anxiety 32

Depression 36

Post-traumatic stress disorder (PTSD) 41

Obsessive-compulsive disorder (OCD) 46

Chapter 2 Staff Training to Raise the Profile of Mental Health in Your School 49

The importance of a mental health initiative 51

Resources on mental wellbeing 51

Supporting a colleague who has been 'signed off' by their GP for their mental ill health 55

Supporting a colleague who is seemingly unaware of their poor mental health 56

Case study 1 58

Additional pressure on staff 63

Case study 2 64

Case study 3 76

Developing staff resilience after an absence due to mental health issues 79

Protecting staff mental health when dealing with safeguarding or mental health issues 80

Staff training 84

Chapter 3 Staff Wellbeing and the Hierarchy of Needs: Staff Wellbeing from the Ground Up 87

Maslow's physiological needs 89

Maslow's safety needs 92

Maslow's belongingness and love needs 95

Maslow's esteem needs 104

Maslow's self-actualization needs 106

Rogers' counselling skills and what they look like in a school setting 107

Chapter 4 Preventative Measures: How to Change Your School Environment to Support Positive Mental Health 111

Workload 111

Marking policy 114

Lesson planning 115

Parents' evenings 117

Email protocols 118

Report writing 120

Behaviour policy 121

Meetings 125

Chapter 5 Activity: Putting the Theory into Practice **127**

Scenarios to explore how to support colleagues 127

Conclusion **133**

Appendix 1: Staff Mental Health Survey Questions 137

Appendix 2: Potential Solutions to Scenarios 141

References 147

About the Author 151

Foreword

It is with great joy that I write the foreword for this excellent book. Joy that the topic is now mainstream enough to warrant the publication of this guide; joy that those who care or are worried will have a practical go-to tool to help them navigate these choppy waters; and joy that my colleague, turned friend, has overcome her imposter syndrome and put pen to paper and fingers to keys and used her personal pain and experience as well as her professional expertise to create something really rather brilliant.

This book is a most welcome addition to the rapidly growing number of books about mental health and wellbeing in education settings because it offers something new and unique. It looks specifically at mental health and illness in staff. A decade ago, student wellbeing was only just stepping out of the shadows of stigma and taboo, a few years later we finally began to think seriously about staff wellbeing and finally, finally with Amy's book we think not only about how to ensure staff are generally happy and well and sufficiently supported and celebrated (still a work in progress) but that those with living experience of mental illness are recognized and supported to do their job well and live their lives to the full.

This matters. This really matters because we know that within any given school there will be numerous staff who sit at somewhere less than 'peachy' on the spectrum of mental health to mental illness. But with recognition, reasonable adjustments and regular reflection these staff can flourish and often become some of our most valued team members and role models.

I care about this a lot because as well as being a professional working in the field of mental health, I also live with a range of mental health issues. I used to hide them. That's just how we used to do things. It almost broke me as a person and certainly meant that professionally I was performing well below par. But things are changing; there have been a quiet army of people like Amy and myself who have been a little more open, a little more honest, a little more challenging of the status quo. Who have, I hope, set the wheels in motion for a more inclusive profession where difference of every kind is supported and celebrated. Where shame and stigma are being actively tackled and where it is okay to seek support and where support is gladly given.

Many people I work with ask me how they can lead a school that is inclusive of staff who face mental health struggles, or how they can support a colleague they are worried about and until now there has never been a specific resource I could point them to.

But now there is.

Thank you, Amy, from the bottom of my heart for writing this book which is a roadmap for the profession as we work our way towards true inclusivity. And thank YOU, the reader, for taking the time to read it and to implement it. The changes may feel small at first; but that's how revolutions start. I promise that within these pages you have everything you need to confidently, sustainably, creatively move towards an environment, culture and ethos that supports all staff, no matter where on the mental health continuum they sit.

Pooky Knightsmith

Mental health advisor, author, speaker and educator

Preface

I have been teaching for 13 years and currently work at a large secondary academy in the South East of England. Having recently reached the grand old age of 34, I have found the courage to do something completely different and step out of my comfort zone to write a book. My hope is that this book will provide practical steps to help schools to be better equipped to deal with the increasing need for staff mental health support. Staff are being asked to juggle more and more balls in an ever-changing and under-funded environment. This is inevitably creating more stress and anxiety, leading to a detrimental effect on teachers' mental health.

During my career, I have worked with many staff who are struggling with their mental health. Depending on where they are on the mental health 'spectrum', they display this in very different ways. Some feel the need to regularly and loudly complain about how busy they are and how hard they are working as a sort of badge of honour that requires admiration. Conversely, I have worked with colleagues who never complain about anything but who have been secretly struggling with serious mental health conditions. Mental ill health can present itself in such a wide variety of symptoms and behaviours that we need to encourage staff to look after each other and take note of any changes in character that could have an underlying cause.

Ultimately, all qualified teachers have a certain innate resilience to even want to teach in the first place, and the teacher training year is probably one of the most stressful in anyone's life. Going into a new work environment with new colleagues can be challenging in itself, without the added pressure of meeting up to 500 new students and having to plan and deliver good lessons day in, day out. Anyone who survives that year must have some protective strategies that have allowed them to qualify. However, a career in teaching is relentless and the levels of pressure rarely decrease; it's just the origin of the pressure that changes. Teachers' mental health armoury needs to be fully stocked with a range of different weapons to protect their mental health. My aim for this book is to give a set of practical 'protective factors' that can minimize the likelihood of staff developing mental ill health.

Despite enjoying being in a school environment as an adult, I spent some of my childhood not wanting to go near school, suffered with severe anxiety and found school a real challenge in many ways. I didn't understand how to make friends, unstructured playtimes and loud activities were a nightmare, and I couldn't cope. I will never forget the extra care, patience and support that many of my teachers showed me. They gave me opportunities to have a quiet, safe space to work during more chaotic parts of the school day, and the education that fundamentally led me to the many wonderful opportunities I have today. This fuelled my passion and drive to support staff in our school community, with a particular focus on their mental health. I am lucky enough to work with many colleagues who regularly go the 'extra mile' for their students, like my teachers did for me. I would hate to think that they might suffer from 'burnout' or even leave such a wonderful profession. If I can, in any way, provide some ideas to keep dedicated and kind teachers in the profession for a little longer during a retention crisis, I will be able to go home with a smile on my face.

I feel the need to explain to you at this point that I have not always got things right with my own mental health, and I am not claiming to be some sort of guru. I have suffered from anxiety which I felt ashamed and scared of, so I kept it hidden from my colleagues and friends until it got to the point that I could not find enough energy to teach in the way that I needed to. I know that you may have picked this book up to read because you are struggling yourself or are worried about a colleague who is struggling. I want to reassure you that disclosing mental health issues is not the end of a teaching career. The courage to be vulnerable means that you will feel more connected to people at a time when your illness makes you feel isolated and alone. You may find that your colleagues are more open to discuss their own mental health struggles, and have just been waiting for the right person to share them with.

Another part of my life is being a carer for my husband who has considerable mental health issues. His experience of employment has been one of ignorance, stigma and even his absence due to mental health issues being mocked. He had to leave his employer due to their inflexibility and lack of understanding of his condition. This delayed him getting the right support and diagnosis for years. I wouldn't want colleagues in any school being subject to these horrific situations and have to leave a career they love and want to continue.

I have been guilty of not looking after my own mental health during the school day. I ran extra after-school revision sessions instead of going to the gym and I chose a quick-grab, unhealthy lunch because I was supporting a crying student. I also did extra work preparing data summaries for Ofsted instead of a catch-up with a close friend and missed a tea break to photocopy resources, and this was all just in one working day. This eventually led me down a slippery slope towards poor mental health and uncontrollable anxiety. I did these things without giving it a second thought, until the point where it cumulatively contributed to me not being able to cope. Many of my colleagues were doing the same and coping, so it became 'the norm', and I felt like a failure for not being able to cope in the same way. I would often attend after-school meetings where it was commonplace to say, 'I must go to the toilet before we start, I haven't been all day' or 'I must have a cup of tea as I haven't had a drink all day.' What I did not consider at the time was that they were not trying to juggle the additional responsibility of being a carer, which can take an emotional toll in itself.

The danger with teaching is that you can get trapped in the 'bubble' of school life, and often it's not until you try to explain the intensity of your day to someone outside of the system that you question its sustainability and effect on mental health.

I am not suggesting that teachers need to become selfish monsters who walk away from crying children and hide in offices, but there must be a balance. Behind the scenes in their bodies things start to take their toll. People choose to work in schools because they want to make sure that children have a safe place to learn and develop, and they want them to be happy. We, as teachers, make sure that pupil wellbeing is at the heart of what we do, and the sight of a new student crying because they are lost or hungry can break our hearts. We know that we may be the positive role models they have in their life, and seeing us each day could be the only positive adult interaction they have. In an average day, we could be supporting a child's mental or physical health or doing something as basic as giving them a clean PE kit or some breakfast. Some of my colleagues deserve some sort of sainthood for the time and care they take changing children's lives and making sure they go home with a smile on their face. However, this often comes at the expense of their own self-care – it can be so easy to forego any hobbies or interests outside of school, which becomes a dangerous case of overworking and never switching off.

Choosing the right people to share your story with is important and it may seem terrifying at the time. However, having to pretend everything is okay when it is not is draining and may exacerbate any existing symptoms. People often feel ashamed of their struggles. As the inspirational Brené Brown says in her book *Daring Greatly* (2012, p.69), 'Shame is the intensely painful feeling or experience of believing that we are flawed and therefore unworthy of love and belonging.' Her TED talks on vulnerability are accessible and can be really uplifting if you are struggling with feelings of isolation due to mental ill health.[1]

I have relied on some wonderful colleagues to help me to regularly prioritize self-care in a way that fits with my personal commitments (by self-care, I don't mean going to a vegan yoga retreat for the week to burn incense or going to a silent retreat for a month – for me, self-care can be going for a swim at the gym, walking on the beach or paddleboarding on the beautiful river where I live). I would like to acknowledge the support of these invaluable people and my husband who puts up with my ever-increasing book collection. He reminds me to look after myself by glaring at me (albeit in a loving way) if I check work emails after a certain time or come up with a mad new school initiative.

My friends have taken me out of my classroom to take off my 'teacher mask' and talk about films, books and other topics that remind me that I do exist as a human outside of the classroom.

---

1 See www.ted.com/talks/brene_brown_the_power_of_vulnerability

Their endless support and love has enabled me to cope with the demands of teaching when I have felt things were too tough to continue. If you are reading this, feeling like you do not have any support, or you are worrying about 'owning your story', I hope that I can give you some practical steps and ideas to put you on the path to recovery and feel empowered to be honest about your struggles.

I have been lucky to work with many inspirational people throughout my career who have been excellent role models for me to look up to and who have led the way for me to reduce the stigma surrounding mental health. They genuinely want the best for the staff they work with and have shown endless time and compassion to colleagues when they have been struggling with their mental health. They were not always experts in mental health, but have spent time learning the best way to support people, and they genuinely care. This has started to change the whole culture in my school, making it a different place to work in compared to many other schools today.

Working in schools can be a truly wonderful vocation that is full of hope. I want people who have committed to the fulfilling task of working with children and making a difference in their lives to be able to carry on being positive about the profession and to swim against the tide of negativity that is being spread in the media. There can be many magical moments during one school day, and there will genuinely be moments when you have the potential to change a student's life with the support you give them. I hope this book gives readers the potential to fall back in love with teaching, if the right support is given.

Introduction

There are already some helpful and important books on general school staff wellbeing. Andrew Cowley's *The Wellbeing Toolkit* (2019) provides a great range of practical ideas to encourage staff wellbeing in schools. Dr Emma Kell's book, *How to Survive in Teaching* (2018), offers a comprehensive and accessible range of ideas to help the teacher retention crisis, but I wanted to write one that explicitly gives guidance on mental health and provides a different set of resources. Mental health and wellbeing are connected because there cannot be a happy school that focuses on just one of the two. The World Health Organization (WHO) defines mental health as 'a state of well-being in which every individual realizes his or her own potential, can cope with the normal stresses of life, can work productively and fruitfully, and is able to make a contribution to her or his community' (WHO 2019).

The fundamental and important difference between mental health and wellbeing is that staff working in schools could have a diagnosed mental health condition but get a tremendous sense of wellbeing from their job due to the support and the way the school adapts to their needs. Conversely, someone without a mental health condition could have low levels of wellbeing. As a document from the Department of Health describes, 'Mental illness and wellbeing are independent dimensions; mental health is not simply the opposite of mental illness. It is possible for someone to have a mental disorder and high levels of wellbeing. It is also possible for someone to have low levels of wellbeing without having a mental disorder' (DH 2014).

There are many other 'invisible' disabilities such as irritable bowel syndrome (IBS) or asthma that may require certain arrangements, and school staff are generally more confident asking for support for these. We have a responsibility to look after our minds as we do our bodies, but we are often not educated about the two equally. In this book I will give an overview of the main mental health conditions that can affect school staff so that there is a common understanding between colleagues about the differences and specific symptoms. It is important to remove the sense of shame in discussions about mental health and to empower people who are struggling to reach out for support.

Why you need to read this book RIGHT NOW!

The UK Government's Health and Safety Executive report from 2018 highlighted the fact that teaching has higher rates of reported work-related stress, depression or anxiety compared to other occupational groups (2100 reported cases per 100,000 for educational professionals, and only 1320 cases for other professions). This clearly shows that there is something quite unique and potent happening in schools compared to other occupations.

The charity Education Support, that offers free 24/7 telephone counselling for all staff working in an educational setting, has reported a huge increase in teachers using their services (Speck 2019a).

Many teachers have used this service at times when they didn't have anyone else to talk to and were suffering from Sunday night back-to-school anxiety. Education Support reported an increase in people contacting them by 28 per cent during 2017–19. The most alarming statistic is that between April 2018 and March 2019, the number of callers assessed as suicidal had increased by 57 per cent on the last year. This equates to 561 people who needed urgent support, which was in most cases as a result of the toxic schools in which they were working. Just let that sickening statistic sink in for a moment before you carry on reading – 561 human beings who were quite probably standing in front of a room of 30+ children the day before, who felt that things had become so unbearable that ending their life was feeling like a viable option.

According to a poll from YouGov for the National Union of Teachers (NUT) in 2015, 53 per cent of teachers were considering leaving the profession (Education Business n.d.). This is a shame and in many cases preventable, with the right support and encouragement. It creates a ripple effect of negativity that may spread to other staff members and affect their mental health too. However, the crisis is not solely about teachers leaving; it is also about recruiting them in the first place. The National Association of Headteachers (NAHT) surveyed a range of primary and secondary school headteachers to ask them about recruitment, and according to the results, 79 per cent said that recruitment was problematic (NAHT 2015). The inability to hire dedicated, qualified staff for posts within schools leads to strains on mental health for the whole school community. Schools are often having to hire teachers who may not be a good choice solely because having someone qualified is cheaper than long-term supply (some supply agencies charge up to £200 per day). This is dangerous because these teachers may be less likely to cope due to their lack of experience or teaching ability, and just leave. This inevitably means that long-term cover and supply has to be hired, which is not good for the mental health of the students or staff in the department. Teaching is a vocation and it relies on teachers giving more of themselves than the hours they are paid for. If this means that as a result staff are neglecting their mental health due to the stresses of hiring low-quality teachers, it is like operating in a pressure cooker and waiting for it to explode.

The more research I did to investigate how mental health affects school staff, the more statistics I found that highlight the urgency of opening up a discussion about mental health in all schools. According to Education Support's *Teacher Wellbeing Index 2018*, 76 per cent of teaching professionals have experienced behavioural, psychological or physical symptoms of stress compared to 60 per cent of all employees nationally. This was linked with the fact that 47 per cent of professionals with mental health symptoms were absent from work for a month or more over the academic year. This staggering statistic is largely due to professionals not feeling comfortable talking about mental health in their workplace, or because they were unaware of the support services that their school could access. Due to national budget cuts, and resources being spread more thinly, teachers are under more pressure than ever before. This can have an adverse effect on staff mental health, and many teachers are leaving the profession as their mental health needs are not being addressed or discussed in their school. Fifty-seven per cent of educational professionals stated that they have considered leaving the profession as a result of health and wellbeing pressures. This is simply not good enough.

Teachers are exposed to stressful events every day due to the contingent and ever-changing nature of their role in school. They are working longer hours than ever before, learning new specifications and working out how to provide for their students with limited resources. Students' behaviour can be unpredictable and erratic, and teachers have to be extremely skilled to manage this, with personalized strategies for each child. All of these factors can take a considerable toll on staff mental health and wellbeing as time for self-care and families is limited. Education Support's *Teacher Wellbeing Index 2019* reports that 49 per cent of staff considered their school culture to have a negative effect on their wellbeing. This means that school staff are more likely to develop mental health issues because their resilience is depleted by the high levels of stress hormones that are released into their body on a daily basis. Without proper support and guidance on mental health, alongside an inclusive programme of wellbeing, things can get very tricky very quickly. This is why we need to talk about mental health in schools RIGHT NOW.

Taking the stigma out of discussions about mental health

Historically, mental illness has been something that society has been ashamed of and kept hidden. The existence of mental asylums in remote locations and lack of discussions within families and communities demonstrates this. The brutal 'treatments' of electric shock therapies and medications with horrific side effects are still recorded in history textbooks and referred to in popular culture. It seems that some adults' reluctance to address and discuss mental health is still partly due to stigma surrounding mental illness. In education, teachers are expected to be strong and resilient in front of their students so that their students feel safe in the classroom. This can lead teachers to carry on pretending that they are happy and then collapsing in floods of tears the moment they get home. Someone I had trained with was working at a school where she was not listened to and felt undermined by her line manager. Her line manager had ignored all her doctor's suggestions for 'reasonable adjustments'. This was having a huge effect on her mental and physical health. She was not sleeping, eating unhealthy food, not exercising and working herself to death to try to earn respect from some pretty nasty-sounding members of the leadership team. She cried most evenings and her relationship with her partner was suffering as she was snappy and distant from him because she didn't want to appear weak. This stopped her getting the right support for her mental health and she had to leave her job because of its cultural attitude (or lack thereof) towards mental health. This should not be happening to good teachers.

Mental health is based on cumulative risk factors that people have experienced in their lives such as bullying, abuse, poverty, disability and physical ill health. Staff will have experiences of some of these factors from the moment that they enter teaching. Their resilience and capacity to adapt to the demands of school life will depend on this. When I use the term 'resilience', I am not suggesting that people with poor mental health have a low resilience by choice, as in they could learn to be more resilient. I mean it is an inbuilt part of their psyche based on their biology and past experiences. This is why all staff members need to be sensitive to their colleagues' past experiences and work out if they may need individual support. It could be that their past experiences have guided their decision to teach in the first place, and that any difficulties could be a huge motivation for them to support children who are going through similar struggles. They look forward to running clubs to support anxious students who struggle to socialize, and will have that extra patience and care when needed because this is either what they had experienced as a child or what they had needed.

Mental ill health is not a choice; it is a complex combination of pre-determined factors that can lead to certain conditions being more likely to occur. The best thing that schools can give to staff is a set of 'protective factors' that act as a buffer. This means giving them the tools and opportunities to practise self-care in a manageable and sustainable way. This book will give staff working in schools some concrete ideas and a range of opportunities to give them as much exposure as possible to these 'protective factors' during the endurance event that is the school year.

Some very experienced and well-educated staff struggle to discuss, acknowledge or manage their own mental health. However, the media seem to expect them to be quasi-counsellors based solely on the fact that they work with children. This is often far from the case as many teachers have come from the toxic 'stiff upper lip' of British expectations. They may have very little knowledge of mental health despite being educated and professional. As everyone has the potential to be at risk from poor mental health, all staff need to receive training, no matter how far into their careers they are. This book will give specific guidance about how to educate staff in a way that is accessible for all.

Unless they have had to support someone living with a mental illness, it is unlikely that staff instinctively know what to say or what to ask as mental health conversations are very different from other conversations. For example, good colleagues help each other with advice and expect to be helped towards a solution and some moral support. With mental health issues, there is unlikely to be a solution in the same way, and incorrect advice may seem patronizing or undermining. This can leave the person feeling unhappy and insecure.

What not to say in response to a colleague's poor mental health:

- 'Everyone feels like this at this time of the school year.'
- 'You could try some yoga.'
- 'Teaching never gets any easier.'
- 'Have you tried thinking more positively?'
- 'We all have bad days.'
- 'What have you got to be depressed about?'
- 'Other people are much worse off.'
- 'Can you stop being so negative?'
- 'You just need to go to bed earlier.'

Within the context of mental health conversations, these could be seen as merely distracting the individual and not listening to the deeper causes behind their symptoms. This could make the person suffering feel belittled, or far worse, it could stop them from sharing their story with professionals and accessing the correct support. Within schools, staff are expected to follow their safeguarding training to support students showing mental ill health, and to some extent they are detached from the situation. It is not easy for staff if the person is a close friend or colleague, and there are often not the same watertight processes for staff mental health in schools. This must change.

Mental ill health has the dangerous power to make people feel worthless, a burden and an inconvenience. It can also lead to intense feelings of isolation and distress, particularly if the person hasn't experienced it before. This, mixed with feeling anxious or scared of things that everyone else seems to cope with and not understanding why, can be a dangerous mix for staff in schools. As Maya Angelou said (1984 [1969]), 'There is no greater agony than bearing an untold story inside you.' According to Education Support's *Teacher Wellbeing Index 2019*, 60 per cent of educational professionals would not feel confident disclosing mental health issues to their employer. This is why destigmatizing conversations about mental health is essential to a mentally healthy school.

If your school culture towards mental health is non-existent and staff are made to feel worthless and weak if they are struggling, something needs to change. Quickly. The modern world of medicine offers many people suffering from mental illness a range of treatment options. It gives them the potential to be happy and fulfilled individuals when the right support is given. This could be through any combination of medication, therapy and lifestyle changes. This means that the associated feelings of shame can be reduced if someone feels brave enough to initiate a dialogue about mental health. There has to be a culture where mental health has been destigmatized so that staff feel as confident talking about it as they would with physical health issues. This is why it needs to start in schools, now.

It is very probable that some staff members may already have extensive personal experience regarding mental health, and might want to join you in planning a strategy moving forwards. There could be a plethora of support in school from colleagues who have previously struggled with their mental health, or who are carers for their partners or other family members suffering from various mental health conditions. They may be waiting for the chance to share their knowledge or experience but were not quite sure how to, or may not yet be ready. Merely opening up a dialogue about mental health in your school and being brave enough to sit with the awkwardness it could bring might be the start of something very exciting and meaningful in your school. It can lead staff members to feel more connected and less ashamed of their different experiences.

Conversations about mental health are hard. They can leave people feeling distressed and upset. Allowing a school culture of not talking about it will lead to staff absence. Good teachers will leave the profession because the right question was not asked due to embarrassment or fear. Many people are afraid they could make things worse by asking about a colleague's mental health, or they worry about saying the wrong thing. School leaders need to be skilled in conversations regarding mental health and this requires them to be respectful of the fact that being honest and vulnerable about mental health issues may be hard and awkward in the short term, but it will be a real investment in staff and could change their future mental health. I will give some suggestions about how staff can be trained successfully to have these conversations appropriately and meaningfully in Chapter 2, on staff training.

This book will hopefully save some time for anyone who wants to start a dialogue about mental health in their school. A cultural change needs to happen at all levels to ensure it permeates throughout school in a sincere and meaningful way. Teaching and working in schools can be a fun, rewarding and exciting vocation. There can be magic and laughter in every day, and you can genuinely make a difference in a child's life. It also has the potential to be all-consuming and detrimental to mental health if self-care is not prioritized. As Eleanor Brown (2013) says, 'Rest and self-care are so important. When you take time to replenish your spirit, it allows you to serve others from the overflow. You cannot serve from an empty vessel.'

Seeing staff as individuals and encouraging self-care

It is explicitly clear that it is not down to teachers to diagnose mental health conditions or attempt to treat them. This is vitally important in maintaining staff's own mental health as the danger is that they may suffer from 'compassion fatigue', which can leave them feeling depressed or anxious as a result of taking on the responsibility of looking after a child's mental health. This is not their job, and must be made explicit from the beginning. However, due to less funding for pastoral staff, teachers have to triage mental health situations on a weekly, if not daily, basis. This is leading to a new strain on the mental health of teachers that could lead them to periods of absence, or worse, leaving the profession entirely. Having two serious child protection disclosures in one day can leave staff feeling completely overwhelmed and tearful. We need to look after and support colleagues as we may not know their backgrounds and how these often horrific and upsetting situations could trigger memories and experiences of their own childhoods. There must be support in place in schools to help staff to cope emotionally after such traumatic situations. I will explain how this can be done in your school later on, when I suggest some ideas for supporting staff in schools when disclosures happen.

Staff mental health and wellbeing must be considered as a fundamental part of whole-school mental health culture. If your teachers are not happy and aware of their mental health, how can you possibly expect them to deliver lessons in which students are happy to learn? As former Education Secretary Damian Hinds said, 'happy, motivated, well-supported teachers are more likely to have happy and motivated pupils.'[1]

In Chapter 1, I explain the main symptoms of the four most common mental health issues affecting teachers. This has been written so that if readers are unsure about certain characteristics of a mental illness they can use the checklists in the first instance to understand more about the conditions and signpost colleagues to the right support. The four most common symptoms are: anxiety, depression, post-traumatic stress disorder (PTSD) and obsessive-compulsive disorder (OCD).

In Chapter 2, dealing with education and training, I explain how staff can be trained in mental health and given guidance to support colleagues and themselves when things feel tricky. In Chapter 3, on work–life balance, I give ideas as to initiatives and policies that schools could put in place to support colleagues. These should be transferable to any school environment irrespective of the age of the students and type of school.

Within each chapter, I give practical advice and case studies of ideas that could be adopted in your school. For example, in Chapter 4 there are suggestions to reduce report writing, and other ideas that may not cost much financially, but cumulatively, they could help staff keep better mental health during the busy school year. In an environment where schools have to manage finances carefully and support staff are being made redundant, all the little 'extra' things that teachers are expected to do soon add up to a tipping point that could lead to 'burnout'.

---

1 See www.gov.uk/government/news/support-on-wellbeing-for-teachers-in-schools-and-colleges

The overall message of this book is of hope, of compassion, and the optimism that everyone working in schools can create and contribute towards a better culture that encourages all staff to talk about mental health, normalize it, and give them the tools to support themselves and their colleagues. It also provides some useful tips and ideas for staff wellbeing. The pressure that school staff face today through funding cuts, specification changes, bigger class sizes and less resources means that they could suffer from 'burnout', leading to good teachers leaving the profession because their mental health is not being supported in the right way, or even worse, because they feel ashamed or unheard.

CHAPTER 1

Common Types of Mental Ill Health among School Staff

According to the Mental Health Foundation, in 2014 12.7 per cent of all absences from the workplace in the UK were due to mental health (ONS 2014). Not prioritizing mental health can cost schools thousands of pounds over the course of an academic year, and not talking about it can lead to further absences, which costs even more money. Inevitably, any long-term sickness of a staff member is very disruptive and stressful for colleagues and students in school, so understanding the key signs of poor mental health can hopefully enable the correct signposting of resources and appropriate support to be put into place quickly.[1]

The key signs to recognize are anxiety, depression, post-traumatic stress disorder (PTSD) and obsessive-compulsive disorder (OCD).

1 The mental health charity Mind has some excellent resources available that can be downloaded and printed for free to use in staff training sessions (Mind n.d., a). The Blurt Project has produced some excellent books and has downloadable resources to use that are extremely user-friendly (www.blurtitout.org).

Anxiety

It is important to recognize anxiety in staff as soon as possible as it can often manifest and cause other types of mental ill health and behaviours such as self-harm, eating disorders, depression, panic attacks or OCD. I will give specific information about the most common of these conditions later on.

Anxiety can manifest as a tricky combination of both physical and mental symptoms. This may mean that it stays hidden behind physical symptoms such as prolonged periods of tiredness, insomnia, sweating, headaches, dizziness, stomach complaints or heart palpitations. It can weaken the immune system by releasing the stress hormone cortisol, which leaves people more exposed to physical illnesses and coughs and colds. If colleagues are suffering from reoccurring poor physical health, it may be worth considering if this is linked to their mental health.

How does anxiety feel?

> *Being a teacher means that to some degree you are expected to have all the answers and be ultra-resilient. However, when I started feeling more nervous than usual about meetings I was expected to attend, I knew that something was wrong. I was feeling physically sick and started to sweat before the meetings and I would spend all day dreading them and considering the worst-case scenarios about them. I felt embarrassed and ashamed that I could not cope with the things I used to look forward to. I couldn't understand why I was feeling like this so I started to isolate myself from my colleagues. My self-esteem plummeted and I was not sure I could cope. Eventually, when I decided to go to my GP and I needed time off to do this, I spoke to the headteacher about how I was feeling. This was terrifying at the time, but being heard and understood made my recovery so much easier. (Susan, age 49, second in charge in English at a secondary school)*

Signs and symptoms

Alongside the distressing physical symptoms anxiety can cause, there are a range of equally worrying thoughts and feelings associated with it. A constant state of worry and feelings of inadequacy and self-doubt can have a massive impact on the ability of school staff to work in their usual way. If your brain is constantly bombarded with worst-case scenarios for day-to-day aspects of your job, and as a result you feel embarrassed and isolated, it can often be easier to phone in sick with a physical complaint rather than risk an awkward conversation with a line manager who has the emotional intelligence of a walnut.

Mind, the mental health charity, has produced a summary of the main psychological and physical symptoms of anxiety (Mind n.d., b).

Effects on your mind:

- Feeling tense, nervous or unable to relax: you may not be able to 'switch off' properly from school and self-care strategies may not provide the usual sense of relaxation. This can lead to delivering poor-quality lessons as you are feeling 'on edge' and are snappy with your students.

- Having a sense of dread, or fearing the worst: this can mean imagining how badly wrong your lessons could go, how you won't be able to control behaviour or any other highly unlikely scenario that may feel scary.

- Feeling like other people can see that you are anxious: avoiding colleagues and interactions, leading to you feeling isolated.

- Worrying that panic attacks might happen: this is a destructive and worrying thought as panic attacks can be scary and are not suitable for a school environment.
- Rumination: thinking a lot about bad experiences and worrying that you have done the wrong thing in response to them.
- Worrying about things that might happen in the future: you spend time and energy worrying about being fired, losing your job through redundancy or your subject being dropped from the curriculum.

Common treatment options

- GPs often ask patients to complete a questionnaire called the General Anxiety Disorder-7 (GAD-7), which measures the severity of anxiety, to determine how to treat it. It may be worth advising a colleague to have a look at a copy online, as this will reassure them that their symptoms are recognized as being part of a treatable health condition rather than something that will last forever.
- There are many self-help resources and workbooks on managing anxiety, and for some people, these will be enough to help them understand and manage their condition. There are online courses available from many providers, and these may be helpful in developing more self-awareness around the issues that could trigger anxiety.

- Some GPs will prescribe SSRIs (selective serotonin reuptake inhibitors) that can be used to help manage the symptoms of anxiety. These are not a quick-fix solution and can take a number of weeks to start working. There are a vast number of different versions available with various possible side effects, so it is important that your colleague has time to attend GP appointments regularly when they are first taking these drugs. GPs may also prescribe beta-blockers to take as a response to specific triggers of anxiety that may occur. For example, if you have uncontrollable anxiety before giving a presentation, then beta-blockers could help to slow your heart rate and alleviate some of your symptoms. These cannot be taken with certain pre-existing conditions such as asthma, however, so they will not be available to everyone.

- Counselling could be used to discuss the causes of anxiety. Again, depending on the availability of NHS counselling services, this is unlikely to happen immediately. It also has the potential to be quite painful and exhausting, so your colleague may need time off to attend appointments and should not have to return to school afterwards when they may not be in a fit state to do so.

- Cognitive behaviour therapy (CBT) could also be used to help make people aware of how they could re-programme existing anxious thoughts and manage them so that they are not so overwhelming and unmanageable.

- Mindfulness-based therapy (MBT) could be used to bring anxious thoughts about the future back into the present moment. The app Headspace is free for educators to subscribe to and has a variety of anxiety-themed meditations to use. Alternatively, the app Calm (which is also free for educators) has various aspects of MBT to help anxiety.

Top three anxiety resources:

- Anxiety UK – if you pay an annual subscription fee to access resources, you get a free annual subscription to the app Headspace included: www.anxietyuk.org.uk
- Clear Fear, a useful CBT-based anxiety resource app that is free to download: www.clearfear.co.uk
- Mind has printable free resources for anything you may wish to know about treatment for anxiety: www.mind.org.uk

Depression

How does depression feel?

> *Depression makes me feel sad. It limits how I can work because it feels like there is a fog around my brain. Everything feels harder than it should. I don't want to talk to people because I feel ashamed and alone. I often feel tearful and I don't get pleasure from the things I usually enjoy. I feel bad for feeling sad because I have a comfortable life and I am very lucky. I feel I cannot be at school when I am like this because my students need a positive role model in their lives. I struggle to do the basics and even getting out of bed and having a shower can seem like a chore. I often struggle to eat healthily when I am feeling depressed and things can seem hopeless. (Danielle, age 32, primary school teacher)*

Signs and symptoms

J.K. Rowling (2016) explained, 'It's so difficult to describe depression to someone who's never been there because it's not sadness.' According to the NHS website there are a range of psychological, physical and social symptoms of depression (NHS n.d., a). The psychological symptoms of depression include:

- Continuous low mood or sadness: this can make teaching impossible as seeing a teacher crying can be unsettling and worrying for students.
- Feeling guilt-ridden: when teachers are expected to be resilient and cope under pressure and they need time off for depression, they can feel extremely guilty and question 'What have I got to be depressed about?' or 'Why can't I cope like everyone else?'
- Having no motivation or interest in things: this can make planning lessons, marking work or even getting up for the day impossible in some situations.
- Finding it difficult to make decisions: this can be particularly tricky if you have a leadership position in a school where people expect you to make quick decisions.
- Not getting any enjoyment out of life: this means neglecting self-care routines and other preventative measures to stop mental ill health.

The physical symptoms of depression include:

- moving or speaking more slowly than usual

- changes in appetite or weight
- unexplained aches and pains
- lack of energy
- disturbed sleep; for example, finding it difficult to fall asleep at night or waking up very early in the morning.

All of these physical symptoms can have a huge impact on your ability to teach. It is such a physically and emotionally demanding role that having a week's worth of poor sleep, poor diet and no energy can quickly turn into a quagmire for depression to invade.

The social symptoms of depression include:

- Not doing well at work: there are so many competing pressures in the school environment to do well that depression will make things harder to manage. Deadlines may be missed and piles of marking could go untouched for weeks.
- Avoiding contact with friends and taking part in fewer social activities and hobbies: having time for social activities is hard to fit in when you are teaching full time anyway. However, when you are low on energy from depression, these things can feel impossible.

Some school staff may have been suffering from depression for most of their adult lives and may not have spoken to anyone at school as they have controlled it with medication and/or counselling. However, if something considerable changes in their lives inside or outside of school, for example the death of a loved one or a close colleague retiring, this could lead to a reoccurrence of the symptoms of their depression and might mean that they begin to struggle to cope at school. Training staff to be confident in both recognizing the symptoms of depression, and having open and honest discussions about how it has affected them, can prevent further episodes becoming unmanageable and leading to staff absence.

Common treatment options

- Lifestyle changes: exercise has been used as a way to help combat the negative thoughts and feelings by releasing the hormones serotonin and dopamine that can improve people's moods. Consider different types of exercise that are available, as maybe the thought of going to a Spandex-based sweaty class could make things worse. Swimming, yoga, Pilates or running offer a more individual approach to exercise that still help to combat the effects of depression. People may also wish to change their diets to include more foods that release vitamins to help fight depression. If you are struggling with depression, reaching out for a quick unhealthy food option can make things worse, so planning your meals carefully can help limit the likelihood of this.

- As with anxiety, some GPs will prescribe SSRIs that can be used to help to manage the symptoms of depression. These are not a quick-fix solution and can take a number of weeks to start working. There are a vast number of different versions available with various possible side effects, so it is important that your colleague has time to attend GP appointments regularly when they are first taking these drugs.

- As with anxiety, counselling could be used to discuss the causes of depression. Again, depending on the availability of NHS counselling services, this is unlikely to happen immediately. It also has the potential to be quite painful and exhausting, so your colleague may need time off to attend appointments and should not have to return to school afterwards when they may not be in a fit state to do so.

- CBT could also be used to help make people aware of how they could re-programme existing depressive thoughts and manage them so that they are not so overwhelming and unmanageable.

- Alternative therapies such as art therapy, eco-therapy and mindfulness could also be useful ways of spending time doing things that can be creative and ease the symptoms of depression.

Top three depression resources:

- Depression UK: https://depressionuk.org
- Mind: www.mind.org.uk
- SANE, Black Dog Campaign: www.sane.org.uk/what_we_do/black_dog

Post-traumatic stress disorder (PTSD)

This mental illness is often incorrectly attributed just to military experiences and traumas caused by the extreme violence of going to war. However, a wide range of different traumatic experiences can lead to the symptoms of PTSD.

How does PTSD feel?

> *I was a victim of a serious physical assault on the way home from school as a teenager. This was really traumatic at the time, but I still get 'flashbacks' of the event as an adult. This means that when I am feeling particularly stressed or anxious I can get a racing heart, be super-sensitive to loud noises and feel 'on edge'. If I witness a violent fight at school it can make me feel really panicky and my body struggles to cope. I struggle to cope in loud busy environments and my body can go into a 'fight or flight response'. (Paul, age 23, primary school teacher)*

Signs and symptoms

According to NHS guidance (NHS n.d., c), several types of events that can lead to PTSD include:

- serious accidents
- physical or sexual assault
- abuse, including childhood or domestic abuse
- exposure to traumatic events at work, including remote exposure

- serious health problems, such as being admitted to intensive care
- childbirth experiences, such as losing a baby
- war and conflict
- or torture.

PTSD is not usually related to situations that are simply upsetting, such as divorce, loss of a job or failing exams. PTSD develops in about one in three people who experience severe trauma (NHS n.d., b). These traumatic events can cause physical and psychological symptoms for many years after the event and can be 'triggered' by certain events in school. As Bessel van der Kolk describes in his text, *The Body Keeps the Score*:

> Long after a traumatic experience is over, it may be reactive at the slightest hint of danger and mobilize disturbed brain circuits and secrete massive amounts of stress hormones. This precipitates unpleasant emotions, intense physical sensations, and impulsive and aggressive actions. These posttraumatic reactions feel incomprehensible and overwhelming. Feeling out of control, survivors of trauma often begin to fear that they are damaged to the core and beyond redemption. (van der Volk 2015, p.2)

This is why people working in schools who have a diagnosis of PTSD need to feel there is someone they can talk to and make them aware of events in school that could trigger a flashback or other distressing symptoms such as a panic attack. For example, if a member of staff has been a victim of sexual abuse in their past, and a student discloses a similar incident, it may illicit a physical response from them and they may need somewhere safe to go to talk about this with a trusted colleague.

Supporting a colleague with PTSD may need to be done by an awareness of their potential triggers and giving them a safe space to discuss any distressing feelings and symptoms that have arisen. This will mean possibly giving the colleague some time away from the classroom and time to use the coping strategies that work for them. It may be doing some exercise, watching a film, painting, listening to music, or something else entirely. They may feel embarrassed by both the original trauma and their response to it, so the fact you have recognized the severity of their experiences will go a long way to ensuring they can come back into work the next day in a mentally fit state.

Symptoms of PTSD include:

- Reliving aspects of the trauma: this could be flashbacks, intrusive images, nightmares, intense distress at reminders of the trauma or physical sensations such as pain, sweating or trembling.

- Alertness or feeling on edge: this could include panicking when reminded of the trauma, being upset or angry, hyper-vigilance, lack of sleep, irritability, being jumpy or self-destructive behaviour.

- Avoiding feelings or memories: feeling like you have to keep busy, avoiding anything that reminds you of the trauma, feeling emotionally numb or cut off from your feelings, being unable to express affection, or using alcohol or drugs to avoid memories.

- Difficult beliefs or feelings: feeling like you can't trust anyone, nowhere is safe, nobody understands, or blaming yourself for what happened.

Common treatment options

- There are lots of self-help resources and workbooks on managing PTSD, and for some people these could be enough to help understand and manage their condition. There are online courses available from many providers and these could be helpful in developing more self-awareness around the issues that could trigger PTSD flashbacks or symptoms.

- Some GPs will prescribe SSRIs that can be used to help to manage the symptoms of anxiety. These are not a quick-fix solution and can take a number of weeks to start working. There are a vast number of different versions available with various possible side effects, so it is important that your colleague has time to attend GPs' appointments regularly when they are first taking these drugs. They may also prescribe beta-blockers to take as a response to specific triggers of anxiety that may occur. For example, if you have uncontrollable anxiety before giving a presentation, then beta-blockers could help to slow your heart rate and alleviate some of your symptoms. These cannot be taken with certain pre-existing conditions such as asthma, however, so they will not be available to everyone.

- Counselling could be used to discuss the causes of PTSD. Again, depending on the availability of NHS counselling services, this is unlikely to happen immediately. It also has the potential to be quite painful and exhausting, so your colleague may need time off to attend appointments and not have to return to school afterwards when they may not be in a fit state to do so.

- CBT could also be used to help make people aware of how they could re-programme existing anxious thoughts and manage them so that they are not so overwhelming and unmanageable.

- MBT could be used to bring anxious thoughts about the future back into the present moment. The app Headspace is free for educators to subscribe to and has a variety of anxiety-themed meditations to use. Alternatively, the app Calm (which is also free for educators) has various aspects of MBT to help PTSD.

Top three PTSD resources:

- Moodjuice self-help guide to post-traumatic stress: www.moodjuice.scot.nhs.uk/posttrauma.asp

- NHS overview on post-traumatic stress disorder (PTSD): www.nhs.uk/conditions/post-traumatic-stress-disorder-ptsd

- PTSD UK: www.ptsduk.org/what-is-ptsd

Obsessive-compulsive disorder (OCD)

How does OCD feel?

> *Living with OCD can feel overwhelming. The intrusive thoughts can make normal life really tricky. It gets much worse when I am feeling anxious already, and the OCD can kick in unexpectedly. I start to repeatedly check taps and switches are turned off in my house. It can take me up to an hour to leave the house as I feel I have to complete my rituals otherwise something bad will happen. I know that the OCD is a symptom for when I feel that things are out of control due to my anxiety. There are certain and routines I do at school to ensure that my classroom is laid out in a particular way. If these things are not sorted, then I feel anxious all day. I have to leave plenty of time to get into school in the mornings in case my OCD is particularly bad. I know I can't be late for work so I get into school early so that I can make sure I have time to check and amend my classroom if needed. I am having counselling to help deal with my anxiety and I have just started taking medication to try to keep my anxiety low enough for my OCD to be managed. (Daisy, age 25, secondary school teacher)*

Signs and symptoms

There are two aspects of OCD that can elicit poor mental health in a colleague. The negative obsessive thoughts can become so overwhelming they can stop a person being able to function generally, let alone be able to teach. The compulsive element of the disorder can also be extremely disruptive to life. If someone is unable to fulfil their compulsions it can cause their bodies to react in the same way as anxiety does. They may start to withdraw from their social lives and personal relationships because they are ashamed or unable to complete their compulsions within certain settings or situations. For example, if someone has a compulsion to check switches repeatedly, this can make going out somewhere public like a cinema or restaurant really tricky or even impossible, as they may not be able to fulfil this compulsion easily. Equally, if they have obsessive thoughts about family members dying if they are unable to complete certain rituals, then if they are unable to complete these rituals, their body will react with a sense of anxiety. This could include symptoms such as a racing heart, sweating, feeling sick or even in its worst case, panic attacks. This can all stop school staff being able to work and can further increase their sense of isolation. Having someone they can speak to honestly about how their mental health is affected by their OCD is really important.

Common treatment options

- People struggling with OCD may be offered treatments such as CBT or medication such as SSRIs. Being able to have time off work to attend appointments or sessions may be needed, so discussing the practical arrangements of this will allow colleagues to feel supported and more in control of the situation. There is a really useful and practical set of guidance on this from the charity Mind on their website (Mind n.d., c).

Top three OCD resources:

- Mind (n.d., c), obsessive-compulsive disorder: www.mind.org.uk/information-support/types-of-mental-health-problems/obsessive-compulsive-disorder-ocd/#.Xbvunrp2tMs
- NHS overview on obsessive-compulsive disorder: www.nhs.uk/conditions/obsessive-compulsive-disorder-ocd
- OCD UK: www.ocduk.org/ocd

CHAPTER 2

Staff Training to Raise the Profile of Mental Health in Your School

When I completed my teacher training in 2007, we were not given any guidance on mental health, either about looking after our own or our students' mental health. If it was ever mentioned, it was in a darkened corner of the staffroom being whispered about. If a colleague was showing signs of depression or anxiety, they were usually told to 'get on with things' or that they would 'get used to the pressure'. They were often reprimanded for their poor attendance rather than anyone trying to identify any underlying causes. When I asked any questions about a particular colleague I suspected may need some support, I was usually told 'they had problems at home' and was encouraged not to discuss it.

Many schools today have a culture of openness and awareness about mental health and have started a meaningful dialogue about it. This wouldn't have been possible without the support of their governors and leadership team. It is not necessarily led by a 'top-down' approach, but encouragement and empowerment of staff to come up with initiatives and ideas. Staff should be offered a range of support that is flexible and appropriate, and looking after staff mental health doesn't always cost schools money (bursars will be pleased about this!). It can be applicable to all school settings if it is delivered in a sincere way by the right people. In this chapter I will suggest ideas for staff training that can allow new teachers to be aware of how to support themselves from the first stages of their career so that it becomes a habit for them.

This will hopefully mean that they do not become one of the many statistics of teachers leaving the profession within the first few years of teaching. More than half of the 9615 cases the Education Support partnership dealt with in 2019 were from staff who had been teaching for less than five years, which doesn't bode well. If staff at the beginning of their careers with fewer responsibilities are struggling with the workload and other stressors of school life, this will add fuel to the fire of the teacher retention crisis. Newly qualified teachers (NQTs) and those who have been working in education for less than five years are 29 per cent more likely to contact Education Support's helpline. This gap between less-experienced and more experienced teachers has widened in recent years alongside reported symptoms such as panic attacks, insomnia, tearfulness and difficulty concentrating (Speck 2019b). Ofsted's recent *Teacher Well-being report* also found that the challenge of retention in the profession is particularly pronounced among teachers who are early into their career: over 20 per cent of new teachers leave the profession within their first two years of teaching and 33 per cent leave within their first five years. Among those with work experience of over five years, there is a more gradual decline – 37 per cent of teachers leave in the first nine years (Ofsted 2019a).

The importance of a mental health initiative

People can be reluctant to change their routines and practices without supporting evidence, and the more cynical staff will potentially disregard a mental health initiative as just another educational 'fad'. Unlike other whole-school initiatives, it doesn't have to be led by the school's leadership team, but it must be supported by them, and led by people in school who care about it. As Simon Sinek argues (2011), if we are trying to implement any successful change within a structure, we must 'start with the why'. Staff will not get on board if you are telling them what they need to do and how to do it without explaining the why first: 'And it all starts from the inside out. It starts with Why' (Sinek 2011, p.39). If you are considering suggesting a new mental health initiative in your school, starting with why it's important will hopefully give you a head start in motivating people to change practice and support your ideas.

Staff mental health has to be prioritized on a daily basis, not just as a token 'Wellbeing Week' to tick a box and make people on the leadership team feel better about themselves. It has to be genuine, well considered and supported by everyone for it to be meaningful and to make a difference.

Resources on mental wellbeing

The Mental Health Foundation has produced an excellent range of resources on supporting all staff with their mental health irrespective of a formal diagnosis of a long-term condition. All members of staff need to be aware of the early symptoms of poor mental health.

Mental Health First Aid (MHFA) England has created various documents that all staff in school could be sent to read, and that could also be given to all new PGCE (Postgraduate Certificate in Education) or SCITT (School-Centred Initial Teacher Training) students working with your school during a training session. It is important that they are aware of their mental health from the beginning of their careers so that it becomes part of their newly established routines as teachers.

The most important part of the document, *Managing Mental Health in the Workplace* (Mental Health Foundation n.d.), that staff could use is a list of signs to spot deteriorating mental health among colleagues. This will enable them to identify certain behaviours, and either have an appropriate conversation with colleagues about mental health, pass it on to the mental health lead, or signpost a colleague to further support if necessary. As teaching is such a highly pressurized and intense role, it is easy for staff to be stressed at particular points of the year when workload is high. However, the symptoms to look out for will often extend past these 'pinch points' and can lead to longer-term mental health issues such as anxiety and depression that may require intervention from a GP or counselling. These could include behavioural symptoms such as missing deadlines or a loss of confidence, but also physical symptoms such as insomnia, headaches or constant tiredness.

'Reasonable adjustments'

Managing Mental Health in the Workplace explains the support that can be offered to staff and 'reasonable adjustments' to help them to be in the workplace after an absence, or to prevent an absence occurring in the first place. These 'reasonable adjustments' are partially taken from the Equality Act 2010, which states that staff suffering from mental ill health should not be disadvantaged due to their condition. This is applicable if their mental health is a long-term condition and diagnosed by a professional (either a GP or psychiatrist).

'Reasonable adjustments' must be manageable and financially viable, however. For example, a full-time paid member of staff could not have reduced hours for a whole academic year. They could have it for a limited period of time, and if their mental health is not improving, then their line manager may suggest a reduction of hours with classes redistributed elsewhere in the school and potentially increasing another part-time colleague's contract. It could be that the colleague has additional responsibilities that are causing mental ill health, so it may be appropriate to have these responsibilities reduced for a short period of time whilst the colleague recovers. It should be made clear that this is to support them, and they will be able to take on more responsibilities in the future. They may need to work from home in their non-contact or planning periods so that they can focus in a quiet environment and have the time to recover from a busy school day. The key part of supporting a colleague by giving 'reasonable adjustments' is that they feel in control of any changes and have time to discuss them face-to-face so that they can ask any questions and plan things with their line manager. 'Reasonable adjustments' are open to being badly handled if email is used to take responsibilities away from staff, making it feel semi-threatening and undermining. I have heard tales of colleagues who have been treated awfully by their line managers when they disclosed a mental health condition. They were made to feel inadequate and powerless at a time when their mental health issues were making them already feel like that.

Staff surveys and preventative conversations

Part of developing a staff mental health strategy or initiative must come from staff themselves. There is no point in the leadership team spending hours in meetings hypothesizing about what would be best for staff. The danger is that people may not feel safe or comfortable talking about their mental health with school leaders, so school leaders may have a distorted view of what is actually going on with their staff in terms of their mental health needs. A good way to address this is through an anonymous staff mental health and wellbeing survey on Survey Monkey, for example (see Appendix 1). This has a mixture of open and closed questions, and feedback from it could be used to create a framework for a mental health strategic plan. It is really important that staff feel listened to and that their needs are met accordingly. Most schools have a wide range of teachers in terms of age and years of experience. Giving them all an opportunity to have all their voices heard to generate individual school priorities is essential. Survey Monkey is an excellent free resource and it saves paper and time, and collates the results for you to analyse via bar charts or pie charts. Although the free version only allows a limited number of questions, it does give the option of adding a comment box to get further information.

The location and content of a mental health conversation is important, and if utilized correctly, it can leave a severely distressed and worried colleague feeling listened to, unashamed, and supported with practical ideas to help their recovery. *Managing Mental Health in the Workplace* (Mental Health Foundation n.d.) also includes useful questions to ask that will aid line managers to work out the correct support and enable the person suffering from mental ill health to reflect on their condition in a safe space. In the survey our school carried out, the other reason that line managers were worried about conversations around mental health was that they thought they would make the situation worse for their colleague or create awkwardness and tension in their working relationship. Again, this could be addressed through staff continuing professional development (CPD) and guidance about what to say and what not to say to colleagues. If schools don't ask staff for their feedback, they won't know this is a problem until a member of staff goes off on long-term sick leave, and by that point it's much harder to deal with and to support them in getting back to work. A preventative conversation can change lives and should be managed well through educated staff.

Supporting a colleague who has been 'signed off' by their GP for their mental ill health

If one of your colleagues is absent from school you might feel awkward about the situation and not be sure about what to say, or conversely, what not to say. Ultimately, your colleague may feel ashamed and upset about their mental health and will need your support. Allowing them to check in with you via their personal email will be appreciated, as being absent from school and missing out on things can lead to more anxiety. This should not be done via school email, however, as it may entice them to do work that could have a detrimental effect on their mental health.

There are some practical things you may need to decide (ideally via a phone call) such as how they want communication with their line manager or Human Resources (HR), where each of their classes are up to (they should not be setting cover work at this time), and how they will contact school about managing their return to work.

Managing their return to work will need to be done in agreement with them, and, to an extent, allow them to be in control of the situation in terms of how much teaching they do on their return (see the case study examples below for 'reasonable adjustments').

Supporting a colleague who is seemingly unaware of their poor mental health

This can be a potentially tricky and awkward situation. You can have colleagues at school who work hard, teach good lessons and volunteer to take on new projects all the time, but you have noticed that their physical health is suffering. They look shattered the moment they come into school, they are not eating during the school day, and they regularly complain of headaches and stomach aches. These ailments have not yet caused absence from school, but a few colleagues have come to you concerned about their wellbeing. They regularly work through their lunch break and have become isolated from their colleagues. They have the classic and toxic British 'stiff upper lip' approach to mental health, and seem unaware that their lack of self-care and workaholism has contributed towards their physical ill health. It is quite possible that they have grown up in a household where mental health was not discussed and may have been seen as a sign of weakness. You know that they live on their own and may not be getting the support they need to look after themselves.

A conversation about their mental health needs to be had by someone, but it has to be the right person. This doesn't necessarily have to be their line manager, but it needs to be someone who genuinely cares, and who can dedicate time to checking in with them on a regular basis, if needed. It could be the first time that anyone has spoken to them about their mental health and they may not recognize their behaviour as damaging their mental health. They may have been waiting for the right person in their lives to ask them the right questions about their feelings. The bottom line is that it must be sincere and the person must feel that they can trust the person they are talking to who will offer support and try to understand their world. As Maya Angelou said, 'I've learned that people will forget what you said, people will forget what you did, but people will never forget how you made them feel.'

If you are the person to talk to a colleague about their mental health, the conversation could be started by showing that you genuinely care about them – something along the lines of, 'I've noticed that you've seemed more tired than usual, is everything okay?' If they say 'Yes, it's fine' in a defensive or dismissive way, at least they know that you care about them and want to help. You could then say, 'I know you've taken on a lot of work recently and I'm worried that you may not have as much time to look after yourself, so if you want to talk to me about any support you might need, please feel free to email me or come to speak to me again.' Having a strong ethos around staff mental wellbeing is important, and information about websites and resources to support mental health should be available in staffrooms. The staff member may go home and think about what you have said and reach out to you for support via email once they've had a chance to think about what you have said to them. It could be that they are too embarrassed or ashamed to have the conversation face-to-face initially. It may be that they ask to meet you to talk somewhere outside of school. Or the conversation could have gone completely over their head and they continue to neglect their mental health until they get to the point of having to take absence from school, in which case, their return-to-work conversation can be the next time to approach the subject. Saying something as explicit as, 'I'm worried about how you are looking after yourself' may then be needed. The worst thing you can do for the person is to ignore the situation or assume their physical health is unconnected to their mental health. The likelihood is that this will lead to further absence and possible 'burnout'.

Case study 1

You have noticed that a colleague is isolating themselves; they are not having their lunch breaks with their usual group of friends and they look tired and tearful in the mornings. They are staying at work later in the evenings and you see them eating more and more unhealthy snacks during the day. They are behind with their report deadlines, which is unlike them, and they have had a couple of recent absences due to 'stomach problems'.

You are due to meet for your normal line management at the end of the next day, so you decide to have a conversation with your colleague about their mental health. It is important to choose a private location, so consider this carefully. Nowadays, many offices (particularly in schools) have a glass panel due to safeguarding requirements, but the ability to have a pull-down blind is needed for private meetings about mental health so you will not be disturbed. The danger of having supportive open-door policies for staff is that they don't respect privacy and pop in to interrupt meetings due to various 'important' reasons. If you have a pull-down blind and it is down, this should deter people who feel the need to call in. It also gives your colleague the opportunity to open up and be listened to, uninterrupted. Also consider the timing of the meeting carefully. If the person is likely to be distressed after the conversation, it may be a good idea to have it at the end of the day so that they can go home and engage in self-care or get further support. Make sure that you do not have another meeting immediately afterwards, so that if you need to contact anyone for support or make notes, you have the space to do this. Make sure that your phone is 'off the hook' and your mobile is on silent so that you are not distracted. After the meeting, it is a good idea to summarize the outcome of it in an email to reassure your colleague that you have listened and have organized the support discussed during the meeting. Actively listen to them in a non-judgemental way and have concrete examples to use as a basis for any conversations. For example, their absences or the fact they have missed deadlines are indicators of poor mental health. It may be the case that your colleague becomes defensive and is not ready to have the conversation at this point, but letting them know that you are there to support them when they are ready is really important. Discussing the possibilities of support that are available to them will give them a chance to think about what they might need. The chances are that they will email you for a meeting at a later date when they have considered the sort of support that may help them.

Ask questions in a genuine and non-accusatory manner, and give them time to talk. A good opening question could be something along the lines of, 'I've noticed that you've been struggling to keep up with deadlines recently. How are you?'

What not to say and do (based on case studies and horror stories from colleagues at various schools):

- Do not have a conversation in the staffroom where others are present.
- Do not try to have the conversation first thing in the morning as they come through the door and are trying to wake up.

- Do not try to squeeze the conversation into a 10-minute window between other meetings.
- Do not take responsibilities away from a staff member without consulting them.
- Do not take classes away from a staff member without consulting them.
- Do not say things like 'Everyone feels sad sometimes', 'Everyone gets stressed', 'Other jobs have longer hours and more stress' or 'You'll get used to the pressure eventually' (yes, these have all been said to colleagues!).
- Do not talk about the mental health of colleagues in a flippant or dismissive way.
- Do not treat mental health less seriously than physical health (the two are often linked).
- Do not tell them to 'think positively'.
- Do not tell them to take up yoga or mindfulness.

It is also important to think about how best to support an emotional colleague. This is crucial because the member of staff is opening up about their feelings and difficulties (and it may even be the first time they have done this with anyone); they will need to feel that you are able to hear this information, listen actively and allow them to 'sit' with these feelings. Unfortunately, some people in schools still think that offering them a tissue and telling them to 'get on with things' is supportive. People cry because they can't cope, not because they want token sympathy and patronizing comments.

When you are having an everyday conversation with a colleague about their weekend plans or the best teaching strategies for a certain student, your brain is assessing how to continue the conversation and link to the topic. You might interrupt accidentally, or you might have things in common and offer practical advice. This can leave you both feeling connected and supported by each other. However, with a conversation about mental health, the opposite feelings could result due to a lack of understanding about what to say. This is why staff need to be trained on active listening strategies.

Active listening strategies:

1. ask open questions
2. summarize
3. reflect
4. clarify
5. encourage
6. react.

Alongside practicalities such as finding a quiet undisturbed location for these conversations, the person leading the conversation must be comfortable listening silently to their colleague. It is important not to interrupt (they may assume you are not listening well), and not to fidget or look at your watch (they may assume you are bored or have a time limit on the conversation). It is also a good idea to make sure your phone is 'off the hook' and your mobile is switched to silent so you are not interrupted at a crucial part of the conversation.

For active listening:

1. It is a good idea to use *open questions* such as 'How have you been feeling?' rather than closed questions that may restrict the information you could gain to help your colleague.

2. After they have explained something to you, it is a good idea to *summarize* what they have said to make sure you have understood correctly. Mental health issues can be complex, and misunderstanding one vital piece of information could mean the difference between a colleague feeling supported or not.

3. It is also a good idea to *reflect* words or phrases that you feel may be significant. For example, if they have said something like 'Things have been tricky recently', it might be a good idea to reflect the word 'tricky' back at them to allow them to consider what they mean by this.

4. Give them time to explain it, to *clarify* a point they have made. For example, if they say, 'I have been feeling unwell recently', it might be appropriate to ask them to explain what they mean by this. It could be physical symptoms linked to mental health, or they may want to talk about their mental health symptoms further.

5. If they are reluctant to talk, small words of *encouragement* could be helpful to allow them to give more details. A simple 'Tell me more' or 'Go on' could encourage valuable information.

6. It is important to *react* appropriately to their information if they have gone through something awful, and it is a good idea to thank them for sharing this information with you.

There is an excellent YouTube video that could be used in a staff training session that goes through these six steps and is based on training from the Samaritans.[1] Even though role-plays can be embarrassing and awkward for adults to do with each other, it is a good idea to get staff to practise active listening to each other talking about something trivial in order to learn and feel comfortable with the various techniques.

Additional pressure on staff

Caring for carers

The *State of Caring* report (Carers UK 2019) highlights that 'the most recent GP Patient survey in England found that carers are more likely to report having a long term condition, disability or illness – 61% of carers compared to 50% of non-carers' (p.21) and that 'carers are seven times more likely to say they are always or often lonely compared with the general population' (p.22). It also showed that 'carers in the UK are nearly twice as anxious as the general population. Carers placed their levels of anxiety at an average of 5.4 out of 10 compared with a population average of 2.9' (p.22). You may be surprised to find out how many of your staff are caring

1 See www.youtube.com/watch?v=oWe_ogA5YCU

for someone alongside their demanding role as a teacher. I cannot overemphasize the importance of building trusting and sincere relationships with colleagues and understanding who is more likely to be at risk of mental health. Working in schools inevitably means you are caring about your students and other staff members, but then having to go home to continue caring for another person can leave carers with little time and energy to complete essential self-care tasks.

Alongside carers, people with physical illnesses or disabilities are at an increased risk. Being absent from school can make you feel isolated and increased feelings of anxiety about going back can make existing mental health issues worse. Teaching is not an easy job to be absent from if this is due to a physical illness, as you are still, in theory, expected to be sending in cover work and contacting your line manager for support. This creates more stress and worry, which can exacerbate any pre-existing conditions. You need to be pro-active in supporting these colleagues and have a bank of cover work so that if they are absent, work is available to collect from staff in school.

Case study 2

One of my colleagues who was the sole carer for her father who had mental health issues told me she was starting to feel uncontrollable anxiety that was exhausting and distressing her as she had not experienced it before. She had recently joined the school's extended leadership team, and this increase in responsibility was the straw that finally broke the camel's back. She had hidden her feelings through overworking and outwardly appearing to be very successful. However, due to her increasingly poor mental health, she could not control a general sense of fear and dread about situations that were unlikely to happen, and did not have the necessary energy to teach for five hours a day.

We spoke about the demands of her caring role that she had kept to herself up until now because it could be quite upsetting and distressing to talk about. I listened carefully and advised her to go to her GP to talk about how she was feeling. This was the first time she had ever been to the doctor's for her mental health, and she was understandably hesitant. We worked out which of her friends could go with her to the appointment for support. Going to get this help can be daunting, which is why it should be discussed carefully with staff as they may not know what to expect. There is an excellent YouTube video from Dr Pooky Knightsmith[2] about which questions might be asked, so I advised her to watch it so that she could think about getting her point across clearly, limiting some anxiety. There is also a YouTube video[3] from the mental health charity Mind, that has excellent resources on their website. When people are suffering from mental ill health, the thought of going to speak to a doctor can be anxiety-provoking and upsetting for them; however, if you follow the guidance from Mind and make a note of how their symptoms have affected them, they can take this with them to their appointment. It could be useful to speak with them about what they would like the outcome of the appointment to be.

Possible questions to consider before your first appointment at the doctor's for mental health:

- How long have you been struggling with your mental health?

---

2 See www.youtube.com/watch?v=PaR-c-tQPTs

3 See www.youtube.com/watch?v=Dqb-n_L5hIA&feature=youtu.be

- Has any major life change happened during this time?
- Which symptoms do you have at the moment?
- How is your diet?
- Do you drink alcohol or use drugs?
- Do you do regular exercise?
- How are you sleeping?
- What do you think could help you?
- Would you like to try counselling?
- Do you think you would like to try medication?
- Are you able to work at the moment?
- Is there a history of mental health conditions in your family?

The time pressures that GPs are under to hit their 10 minutes per patient quota means that the conversation may feel rushed, so your colleague could ask the receptionist for a longer appointment. If someone is at the point of not being able to go into their workplace due to their mental ill health, GPs can give them a medical certificate and suggest lifestyle changes before offering counselling or medication.

Depending on where you live in the country, the waiting list for

NHS counselling sessions is as long as six months, so it may be worth investigating if your school has links to a free counselling service that staff can access more quickly. The NHS usually offers a maximum of six sessions and the availability of counsellors can be quite restricted. The telephone counselling services offered by some organizations such as Education Support could be more accessed more quickly and may be more suitable for some people. Alternatively, your academy chain or county council may have invested in counselling services to support staff. If they are thinking about medication, Mind has some fantastic resources that may answer any questions colleagues have about side effects or dosages. It also suggests alternatives to medication such as exercise, mindfulness, diet and art therapy.

Medication for mental health conditions usually takes 4–6 weeks to start working as the body adapts to them, so they are not a quick fix. If colleagues start medication, it is a good idea to encourage them to tell their line manager so that they are aware and can support them if they are suffering from any side effects. Depending on the type of drug, side effects may include things like weight gain, sleeplessness, tiredness, headaches or upset stomachs, none of which will make teaching seem easy or manageable. These side effects usually start quite soon after taking the drugs, although after a week or so they should ease and make things easier to cope with.

Education Support has a free 24-hour counselling service for all educational professionals that may also be useful if colleagues need advice or support at a random time. Insomnia is often a product of poor mental health, so having someone to talk to at 2am may be needed. If staff need time off school to attend counselling appointments, this needs to be considered carefully. If the counselling sessions have been distressing (which inevitably they can be) and the member of staff wishes to come back into school afterwards, it may be a good idea for them to have someone to check in with before they start teaching. They could be in a fragile emotional state and the demands of teaching 30 hormonal teenagers for an hour could simply be too much. It is important to allow them to decide what they think is best for them, unless you have reason to doubt their judgement based on prior situations. Then, it may be important for you to make the decision for them in a caring and supportive way. They may like the routine and safety of being in the classroom, and find it more beneficial to come back after a session to teach as missing a lesson may be more stressful for them. However, it is best for everyone if they have their line manager or member of the senior team available on their return to assess the situation and show they care and can help if needed.

On return from the doctors my colleague was given a medical certificate for a phased return to work and reduced duties. We met first thing the following morning to go through the plan for her week ahead. At this point any extra interaction with people was a real stress to her, and she simply did not have the energy to teach a five-lesson day as the constant worry about things was draining. First of all, we went through her exam classes and worked out if she could continue with these as they are intrinsically more pressurized than other lessons. She said at this point that she was happy to continue teaching them, but would let me know if it got too much. We then went through days when she was due to have no free periods, and I suggested she went home at lunchtime on those days so that she could rest or go for a walk to get some fresh air or exercise. This would give her time to build her reserves back up and work out how much she was able to do the following week. We met each week on a Friday morning to go through the plan for the following week so she had less anxiety over the weekend worrying about what she could or could not do.

I also referred her to Occupational Health to discuss how her anxiety was affecting her at work. Other colleagues have said that they are really reassuring, and because they are an independent service, they can be trusted to do what is best for you. During the appointment she went through a list of things that triggered her anxiety, and this was really helpful because it meant we could go through the report together and come up with a care plan (see the examples below). We wrote a list of things that she felt comfortable doing and things that she found tricky at that point. This was so helpful for us both to do together and go through the specifics. For example, going to a course at a new school was too much for her anxiety to cope with, whereas doing parents' evenings (with a scheduled break in a quiet room) was an option. The loudness and brightness of the big sports hall with all the other conversations going on was too much, but opening the room up next to it made it manageable and she could cope. This saved her the anxiety of the previous week worrying about whether she would have a panic attack in front of the whole room of staff and parents.

The care plan we came up with went through the signs that indicate her mental health was deteriorating, what to do if anyone noticed these signs, what she was happy to share (and who with), situations in school that caused her anxiety and a self-care plan in school of things that would keep her well.

If something had happened during the day that had made her more anxious or worried, she could email me in the evening after school rather than see me face-to-face. I would always reply with a practical solution and the option of discussing it further, if needed. Knowing that someone was taking the time to care and make sure she felt supported made such a difference in her recovery.

Certain aspects of her role were changed to limit the amount of exposure to anxiety she would have to deal with, and she would be reducing her hours slightly the following year so that she could continue to do things to look after her mental health.

This case is not unique, and different care plans can be put in place depending on the needs of the staff member. However, this is not always the case. There are still schools that ignore GP medical certificates, refuse to address mental health concerns about their staff, and do not feel it's important to put support in place or offer staff a chance to talk about their mental health. This leads to good teachers leaving the profession as their self-esteem hits rock bottom and they do not have the capacity to deal with such a big thing on their own. A care plan could be used to give clear guidance about the support a colleague may need and would want if they are struggling with mental ill health.

Care plan example 1

Signs my mental health is deteriorating:

- taking on extra work or projects
- avoiding talking to people at breaks or lunchtime
- making jokes to deflect from how i'm feeling
- not socializing with my friends outside of work
- not exercising or talking about plans to exercise
- being quiet and avoiding eye contact

- deflecting any conversations that may involve talking about my feelings or home life
- not wanting to go to meetings with large numbers of people (e.g. staff briefings).

Physical signs:

- poor management of diabetes
- tiredness
- racing heart.

If you notice these things are happening and you are concerned, please do the following:

- Ask to speak to me about it at the end of the school day in a private, undisturbed location. I am happy to talk about my mental health with people I trust.
- Speak to my line manager about your concerns if you are not sure what to say to me.

What I am happy to share:

- I have been experiencing symptoms of anxiety. I am a carer for my husband who has significant mental health issues and may not be capable of looking after me sometimes. I have not had counselling yet, but I am due to start soon. I have not been on medication in the past and I am not on it currently. I can find it hard to express or process emotions so may need some quiet time to talk to someone after something has triggered my anxiety.

Situations in school that may trigger my anxiety are:

- situations where I don't feel in control (e.g. watching a fight happen in school)
- feeling trapped in a meeting with lots of people
- not being able to contact my husband
- places with loud background noise or bright lights (being in the hall for parents' evenings)
- feeling physically tired from lots of social interaction (like parents' evenings)
- being emotionally drained from my role as a carer (after attending appointments with my husband)
- coming back to school after a holiday
- (the possibility of other situations I am not currently aware of).

Self-care plan in school:

- sit by the door in meetings in case I feel I need to leave

- give my husband's phone number to my friends in school in case my phone breaks
- have lunch outside my classroom with a friend
- talk about any uncomfortable feelings with someone I trust
- message my line manager in the morning if there is something that could affect my teaching for the day or if I need last-minute cover
- ask my head of faculty for support with specific lessons if needed
- 'check in' about my mental health as part of line management meetings each fortnight, even if I don't immediately bring it up.

Another example was for a member of staff who has been suffering from depression since their teenage years. They have had various successes with medication and counselling in the past, and enjoy their job. They have a proven record of good results and have added lots of resources to the department. They really care about the students and enjoy supporting extra-curricular trips, taking them to various places to develop their learning further. However, their elderly father has become increasingly ill and they are having to spend more time looking after him. This is having an impact on their mental health and their symptoms of depression have re-emerged. This is an example of their care plan.

Care plan example 2

Signs my mental health is deteriorating:

- I gain weight as I binge-eat unhealthy food.
- I don't do any exercise.
- I isolate myself and avoid busy situations like staffrooms.
- I stop attending meetings because I can't cope.
- I miss marking deadlines.
- I get snappy with colleagues.
- I find it hard to sleep.
- I am tearful at things that should not make me tearful.

If you notice these things are happening and you are concerned, please do the following:

- Ask to speak to me about it at the end of the school day in a private, undisturbed location. I am happy to talk about my mental health with people I trust.
- Speak to my line manager about your concerns if you are not sure what to say to me.
- Do not avoid talking to me in case you upset me.

What I am happy to share:

- I have suffered from depression since I was a teenager. I am currently receiving counselling and am taking medication to support my mood. If I am upset and tearful, please don't ignore me. Feel free to keep making jokes around me and talking about the usual things. I usually binge-eat if I am feeling depressed and I'm not always aware of this, so feel free to remind me quietly about the importance of trying to eat healthily. Even if I am unable to teach due to my mental health, the routine of getting up, dressed and being in school is better for me than staying at home.

Situations that might trigger my depression:

- stressful behaviour situations at school
- busy marking periods during the year
- my health becoming poor
- my family's health deteriorating
- gaining weight
- not being able to exercise.

Self-care plan in school:

- messaging my line manager if my mood is deteriorating to the point I am tearful and cannot sleep

- having a quiet office I can work in on my own if needed
- doing regular exercise
- eating healthily
- socializing with friends in the pub on a Friday after school
- reading somewhere if I need some time out.

Case study 3

This support staff member had suffered from depression and anxiety since her teenage years. A change in her role at school had meant that she was suffering from long periods of depression and was feeling anxious on a daily basis. She has been back to her GP about restarting her medication. At work, during a lesson, she suffered from a panic attack and had to leave the room. Her GP subsequently signed her off from work for two weeks, with a phased return.

Care plan example 3

What are the signs to look out for that my mental health might be deteriorating?

- irritability, aggression, tearfulness, swearing profusely when venting
- being withdrawn and not participating in conversations or out-of-work activities

- inability to concentrate
- restlessness
- indecision
- difficulty remembering things or losing train of thought when talking
- loss of confidence
- struggling to tolerate other people
- taking on too much work or saying yes to projects
- being louder than usual
- listening to music via headphones in the faculty office to shut out background noise.

Physical signs might include the following:

- constant tiredness
- headaches
- complaining about waking early and not sleeping
- weight loss or gain
- IBS getting worse and not being managed.

If you notice these things are happening and you are concerned, please do the following:

- Talk to me in the first instance about your concerns, but please make time for this conversation so I am not rushed and can process things.
- Speak to my line manager if you do not feel you can speak directly to me.
- If you have real concerns about my mental health and do not feel I should be at work, contact my partner [insert name and phone number here].
- It helps me if people tell me that they can see that I'm struggling as I find it hard to start the conversation and to ask for help and support.
- Find a quiet place for me to be.

What I am happy to share:

- I am happy for colleagues to know that I suffer from anxiety and depression, and I am happy to discuss this with them.

Self-care plan for in school:

- have lunch every day (preferably outside, in a quiet space)
- a point of contact in case I feel anxious or feel a panic attack coming on

- being able to get some headspace during busy days
- being able to use headphones to distance myself and get some downtime
- meet fortnightly with my line manager so I can review how things are going and reflect.

Developing staff resilience after an absence due to mental health issues

Once staff have been honest about their mental health issues and have returned from a period of absence, this time is crucial and could determine how their recovery continues. The ability to have regular check-ins with someone they trust is vital. It won't always be their line manager, but it needs to be someone on the senior team who can organize cover if needed. Ultimately, as people are recovering, they may feel able to do more and more of the things that had caused them anxiety and build up to taking on more teaching and more responsibility, but this must be done gradually, in a supported and manageable way.

If someone suffering from mental ill health feels out of control from the symptoms of the condition, the worst thing to do is to force them to take on more than they are able to. Helping them to build their confidence and resilience is vital and can ultimately aid their recovery. If they need to have time off to go to counselling during the school day, it may not be possible for them to return to school afterwards, so you should factor this in. Alternatively, if they have evening counselling sessions, they may need to check in with someone the following morning to make sure they are emotionally capable of teaching and are managing to cope with the process.

If someone has been through a trauma and has to relive it through counselling, this can be emotionally draining and may mean that the staff member is not able to 'play the part' of a teacher for the whole day following this. It might be that they want to come into school to be around others and work in a quiet office, but not be able to teach. Making this 'reasonable adjustment' for people will be rewarded in the future when they have finished counselling and made progress with their mental health. It makes them feel valued and cared for when they are at their most vulnerable, and school may be the most stable and consistent place in their lives if they have no one to care for them at home (which is surprisingly common, despite people having families or partners). It might be that they have not disclosed to their families that they are struggling with their mental health at all, so school provides a vital component of their recovery, and providing the right environment to talk about mental health is crucial to that.

Protecting staff mental health when dealing with safeguarding or mental health issues

The term 'compassion fatigue' was originally applied to nurses during the 1950s who were becoming less compassionate towards their patients due to the secondary trauma stress they were experiencing from the relentless nature of looking after others on a daily basis. Today, it is still referred to as secondary trauma stress when teachers show signs such as increased irritability with students, decreased concentration and dreams about a student's own trauma. Teachers are frequently exposed to potentially distressing and upsetting issues as part of their ever-increasing list of responsibilities. This isn't a bad thing in itself as it means the children feel they have someone to trust in school, and due to media exposure about child abuse, they are more confident in reporting it. However, classroom teachers and support staff are often put in a disclosure situation where students are coming to them with pastoral issues that are distressing in nature, and these have the potential to be upsetting and 'triggering' for the staff member.

The UK Government announced that this is the first time that a group made up of mental health professionals and education staff have worked together in this way. Schools minister Nick Gibb added:

> One thing that strikes me when I meet teachers in every school is their selflessness and their willingness to go above and beyond to help their pupils. However, like any important and rewarding job, life as a teacher brings its own challenges and pressures. I saw first-hand the crucial role this group will play in providing us with expert advice to help prioritize teachers' mental health and wellbeing – setting a positive example for pupils. (quoted in Belgutay 2019)

It seems that the term 'selfless' in his quote intends to show teachers in a positive light. However, Gibb is underestimating the danger of losing one's 'self' through consistently putting others' needs before their own. Teachers' selflessness can take its toll on mental health if not managed carefully. Teachers can easily be exploited by this unrealistic ideal of 'selflessness'. If they do not set careful boundaries for themselves, they risk neglecting their mental health to the point that their ability to teach well is compromised.

If this is not managed carefully by the staff themselves and the leadership team, it could lead to 'compassion fatigue' in staff, which can create a negative culture and poor mental health in pastoral staff who are having these conversations more and more regularly. With funding for external services being reduced by UK Government spending reductions, children have to disclose their mental health to teaching staff as there are very few groups operating in communities who can help them. Although Child and Adolescent Mental Health Services (CAMHS) has different tiered systems to prioritize certain cases, most children will not meet the threshold for treatment, so it is often left to schools to provide psychologically for the child on a day-to-day basis. The '*2018 CAMHS Project*' found that the average waiting time until the first assessment for a child was 9 weeks, and the average waiting time for the start of treatment can be 13 weeks (NHS Benchmarking Network 2018). This means that schools are having to manage and support children with potentially very poor mental health, and staff are expected to absorb the emotional strain of this. A child who is tearful every day, self-harming and suffering from an undiagnosed eating disorder will still be in school trying to learn and do their best. The reality of this for the member of staff to whom they have disclosed can be exhausting and relentless.

The Ofsted *Teacher Well-being* report (2019a, p.31) found that 'respondents reported that funding cuts have reduced access to external specialist support. This results in staff taking on extra responsibilities outside of their area of expertise, which adds to workload and pressure: "Teachers have to support pupils with some really serious home issues. It is emotionally draining... Pressures caused by limited wider resources e.g. behavioural support, educational psychologists".'

In other professions, such as care homes and counselling, staff have supervision, which allows them to have the time to reflect and process uncomfortable and distressing feelings that have arisen from a mental health disclosure. Often schools just expect staff to carry on, do the relevant safeguarding process for their school, but rarely follow up on the staff member who has been involved. In Nathalie Downing's *Tes* article, 'Wellbeing: Why don't schools offer staff supervision?' (2019), she wrote: 'Often emotionally intense professions such as social work, offer safe spaces to offload, yet the practice is almost unheard of in schools.' She explains how, after 20 years of teaching, she would find herself crying in a layby after an emotionally tough day. She asks, 'Where do we empty our emotional buckets? Where does all this messy stuff get discharged? I know what most of us do with it: try to bury it and ignore it. Or eat it. Or run if off.' This is simply not good enough and can lead to staff suffering from mental and physical ill health and subsequent absences. It can also lead to a relapse in staff members' mental health if they are suffering from PTSD and a child has unintentionally encouraged them to relive their own traumatic experiences by how the child has described them. In schools there must be a genuine desire to care for staff and allow them the time and space if it is needed. In the majority of cases it will not be used, but staff need the reassurance of knowing that it exists if need be. If a child has made an upsetting disclosure and staff are affected emotionally, senior team members should be available to cover lessons if necessary, and give staff the space and time to discuss how or why it has affected them in a certain way. This shows the member of staff that you genuinely care about their mental wellbeing and are prepared to accept the impact that such distressing disclosures can have on them. It also helps to eliminate any shame the staff member may have if the disclosure brings up personal feelings. It can allow the correct support to be put in place if a similar incident happens in the future, and allows them to feel heard and understood, rather than alone and ashamed. As Brené Brown says in her TED talk 'Listening to shame', 'If we share our story with someone who responds with empathy and understanding, shame can't survive.'[4] In schools, there must be someone who can be trusted to offload to after a mental health disclosure from a child.

Staff training

Mental health initiatives for staff are really important and should not be the sole responsibility of the senior leadership team or staff. It must be a genuine and considered approach that allows all staff to feel comfortable talking to someone about any mental health concerns they have. In our school, we have 12 trained Mental Health First Aiders – a group carefully selected from a wide range of positions within the school did a two-day Mental Health Foundation training qualification. It was important that this group was made up of approachable people who were ideally spread across the school site. The training course went through all the signs and symptoms to look for mental ill health in students, although these were also applicable to staff. The group explained their roles during a Monday morning staff briefing, and were there to support staff if needed.

Ultimately, you need as many staff to be trained about mental health so that every single member of your staff has someone they trust to go to for genuine support. There are often horror stories about line managers using mental ill health against their staff, and not knowing what to say or do. This makes the already stressful situation worse and could lead to long-term staff absence. There needs to be a range of staff who are trained so that staff can choose the right person for them. It could be a colleague, a line manager,

---

4 See www.youtube.com/watch?v=psN1DORYYV0

a member of the leadership team or support staff. Their title is irrelevant for conversations about mental health; they just have to have a caring personality and be trained to ask the right questions and signpost to the appropriate resources. Supporting this, there must be an official referral system if staff are worried about a colleague's mental health and are not sure about how to have a conversation with them about it, or if they have been upset about a colleague's disclosure, and might need support themselves. This needs to be a trusted member of the leadership team who has been trained and has the authority within the school to make changes to support the colleague who is struggling. When I say trusted, I don't mean that they will keep the mental ill health of a colleague a secret; I mean that they can be trusted to discreetly do the right thing to support them. One of my ex-colleagues who was absent with anxiety told me that they felt isolated in their faculty area of the school and did not want to speak to their line manager about such a personal thing. This is why all members of staff need to have access to a wide range of opportunities and the space to be listened to, if needed.

Leadership teams could have an open-door policy to allow staff to drop in to speak to them on the way into school, during breaks and lunchtimes, and after school, if needed. This reassures staff that they can speak to someone if they are suffering from things that affect their mental health, and makes them feel cared for. Having the option of popping in to have the space to be heard can be particularly important if the member of staff lives on their own or does not have someone at home they can speak to. We may assume that adults have a wealth of friends they can talk to about their mental health, when in reality there are many staff members who could be too ashamed or embarrassed to talk to their partners or family about their illness. Having someone impartial who can listen to their concerns without judgement is vital, and sometimes it may not initially feel appropriate to have the conversation with friends or family.

CHAPTER 3

Staff Wellbeing and the Hierarchy of Needs

Staff Wellbeing from the Ground Up

Abraham Maslow first published his 'hierarchy of needs' in 1943 in his paper, 'A theory of human motivation'. It was an attempt to work out the different aspects of the human experience that lead us to be happy and fulfilled individuals. It combines physical and psychological needs as part of a hierarchical structure that starts at more basic physiological needs and moves to the aim of self-actualization, where the person can become the best they can be.

Many different counselling approaches today use this hierarchy as a way for clients to develop their self-awareness and to move forward with their lives. Carl Rogers developed the humanistic or person-centred approach to counselling from the 1940s onwards. He used Maslow's hierarchy as a foundation to establish a modality of counselling that aims to support people experiencing mental ill health.

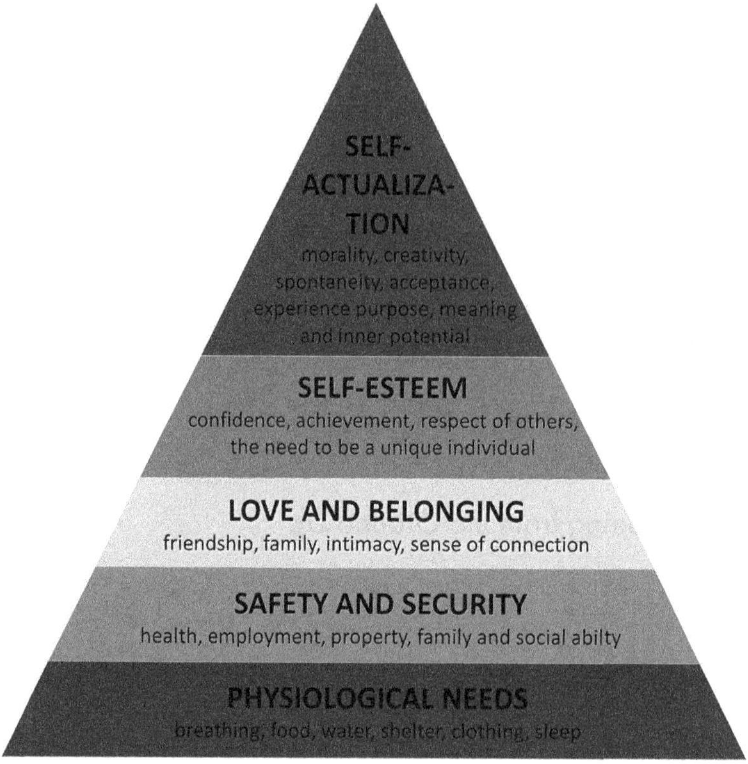

He argued that in order for people to reach the self-actualizing layer of fulfilment on Maslow's hierarchy, the counselling process needed to have three main conditions. These should be something that schools aspire to have in some form in order for all staff to flourish and to live up to their potential. The first condition is the idea of listening non-judgementally, which Rogers called 'unconditional positive regard'. The second is listening with empathy and trying to understand how it feels to be in the other person's experiences. The third is known as congruence, which is the idea that the person listening must be authentic and genuine in their interest. They must want to support and help, rather than pretend to, or because they have to listen as part of their job.

If schools can facilitate these conditions in some way, or provide a service that does this, the colleague struggling with their mental health will be able to reflect on their needs and be on the road to recovery. Line managers should not aim to be counsellors for staff as they will not have the formal supervision processes to protect themselves from any potential issues this could raise for them. Perhaps using Rogers' therapeutic components in conversations about mental health could be used to structure some practical solutions to support colleagues.

When it comes to looking after the wellbeing of staff it may be useful to consider how the various aspects of Maslow's hierarchy of needs can be applied to staff working in schools alongside the conditions for a supportive conversation about mental health.

Maslow's physiological needs

Ideas to fulfil the food and drink needs of staff

- Offer tea and coffee making facilities in Monday morning briefings or meetings.
- At the start of the new school year on the first day back, lunch could be provided.
- Before evening school events there could be the option of having free sandwiches, cake and fruit.
- At Christmas, there could be a charity staff-cooked breakfast on the last day of term.
- On sports day, where staff may be asked to run an event in

the sunshine, students who cannot participate could make cakes that are then delivered to staff by pupils as they are 'scoring' the different events.

- Offer staff a Fruity Friday at the end of the week in the staffroom to give everyone a treat at the end of a busy school week.
- Have a staff version of the *Great British Bake Off*, which can really help to raise staff morale during the dark winter months. The competitive element and choosing your own version of Mary Berry and Paul Hollywood to be the judges works well (their face masks are available to buy online to make things feel more authentic).

Remember to include different dietary requirements such as gluten-free or vegan, as you want these ideas to be inclusive to all.

Food and drink needs in action

After a whole-school staff training session on mental health and wellbeing, staff were asked to write down improvements for staff wellbeing in our school. It was really important that we were genuinely listening to staff ideas so they felt cared for and supported. The training session had been quite heavy in terms of discussing self-harm, suicide and depression. I was expecting some deep and meaningful responses, such as free counselling services for staff; however, on every mind map of ideas one feature was common – more milk.

We have a main staffroom that contains the milk that is delivered, as well as lots of faculty offices, where people usually spend their breaks and lunches. It had become common practice on a Monday morning for the designated 'milk monitor' for the faculty to collect a bottle on their way into work, but this was leaving the main staffroom depleted. Our school budget was decreasing, so we just needed to be smarter with it. The next day, I came into school, and an unnamed individual had come up with a solution to the staffroom milk problem. They had attached a four-pint bottle to the door of the fridge with a metal, yes, metal, chain, so it could not be removed. Despite staff members chuckling about this idea when they went to pop their lunches for the day in the fridge, it made me reflect on Maslow's hierarchy of needs and how schools can address this, starting from the basic needs level. It is a good idea to have tea, coffee, squash and sugar in your communal staffroom readily available and free for all staff. This is important as it creates less stress in a back-to-back teaching day. It also shows staff that you care about their basic needs. Not being able to make a cup of tea or coffee when needed could be the straw that breaks the camel's back, so to speak.

The mental wellbeing of new mothers and fathers

Another part of Maslow's hierarchy covers the conditions to reproduce happily, which means being able to have children and have mental health support if needed on a parent's return to school. Schools must support and discuss the mental health of new mothers. Post-natal depression (PND) affects 1 in 10 women and can surprisingly occur up to a year after the birth of a child. This means that if a woman returns to work before her child's first birthday, she may be at risk. The signs and symptoms of PND are similar to depression (as outlined previously). Similarly, new mothers' partners could be struggling with their mental health due to the arrival of a new baby causing extra worry and anxiety in their lives. Schools offer 'Keeping in touch' days for women returning to work to come back into school, prepare resources, meet with staff and prepare psychologically to return. During these days it is a good idea to ask returning colleagues about their feelings regarding returning to work, the support they have, their mental health and any support they might need. For example, they may request to finish early so that they can pick their children up from school, or other 'reasonable adjustments'. Another option is for mothers to have a phased return to work when they carry out a partial timetable for a set number of weeks. This will help them readjust to the busy demands of school life. These support strategies should also be available for new mothers who are adopting children into their family, or fathers returning from paternity leave.

Maslow's safety needs

Suggestions for healthy bodies, healthy minds

- Visiting an on-site beauty therapist (they could visit during the school day, so that staff can have their manicures or pedicures during a teaching period).

- Give all staff free access to the school fitness suite that staff can use before or after school. (It may be useful to consider a staff-only session for self-conscious staff members who don't want to flop any wobbly bits about in front of students.)

- Organize a nurse to come in to school to do flu jabs to help keep staff well so that they don't have to try to fit the time into their busy routines to get it done elsewhere. Some headteachers choose to pay for all members of staff to have the jab as a way of showing they care about staff.

- Organize a free yoga or relaxation session for staff after school each week.

The key to staff physical wellbeing is a bit like differentiation in teaching – you cannot have a one-size-fits-all approach – it has to be personalized and appropriate.

Communication about change

Change can have a disproportionate effect on staff members who are suffering from mental ill health. In a climate of budget cuts and redundancies, staff can feel that their jobs are no longer safe when things change. According to Education Support's *Teacher Wellbeing Index 2018*, 30 per cent of staff considering leaving teaching due to their mental health stated that rapid or organizational change was the main reason for this. Regular communication from the leadership team is important so that staff feel involved with any changes to workload during the year. Do not underestimate the impact of large-scale changes such as moving classroom locations for staff, or small-scale changes such as a different system on which to take registers.

People with mental ill health could have less resilience to change and will therefore need as much warning as possible about any changes to their routine. Part of their recovery and continued management of their condition could be reliant on the fact that they have certain rituals and processes that they anchor themselves on. Knowing your staff and colleagues will enable you to identify who may need extra support during periods of change. Their behaviour may present as resistance to change, but this could be a defensive strategy because they are scared rather than because they disagree with the change. Understanding this can allow colleagues to have a quiet conversation after a meeting to find out about their worries and to listen, instead of assuming that they are trying to launch a mass rebellion or uprising against the system.

The Ofsted *Teacher Well-being* report (2019a, p.7) concluded that, 'Educators told us that they do not have enough influence over policy, which changes too quickly. The impact of that is experienced as negative for two main reasons: frequent changes increase the already high workload; and the perceived lack of say leads to feelings of de-professionalism.' Our middle leadership team, made up of all heads of department, pastoral leaders and the senior leadership team, meet once a half-term to review policies, discuss priorities and discuss any changes to workload so that staff have the opportunity to feel heard and that any changes have been well considered by all stakeholders.

As an example, when schools introduce a new online rewards and behaviour system, it could be presented during a meeting, and staff could be given the opportunity to ask questions and to test it out in practice. This will mean that by the time it is presented to staff in a training session, most people in the room will have already practised using it and could save stress by helping other less computer-confident staff out.

Having weekly briefings on a Monday allows staff to highlight and discuss any events coming up in school such as visitors and priorities for the week. It is good for everyone to be brought together like this, and makes people feel like they are aware of things that may affect their workload.

Change is an inevitable part of working in a huge system of policies and processes, and schools are under huge pressure from the UK Government or their academy chains to move things forwards. However, the management of this and the consideration of people during this change is vital for staff suffering from mental health conditions. A quiet conversation with them prior to a meeting could be the difference between them processing the change and working out how to cope, or them going home in floods of tears and being absent.

Maslow's belongingness and love needs

How to create a genuine sense of staff wellbeing activities in your school

Ultimately, supporting the mental health of your staff does not have to cost a lot of money, and if you ask staff for ideas and support, you are bound to get a team of people who care about mental health together to run activities or events. People like to feel they belong to a school community that cares about them, and this care needs to come from all levels and positions so that all members of staff feel supported. If they know that they have a supportive line manager who genuinely cares about staff wellbeing, and know you well enough that you are able to spot early warning signs, then they are more likely to open up and be honest about any mental health issues. People generally need to know there is someone they trust who they can go to when things start to go wrong, and they need support. This may not be their line manager, but hopefully if all leaders are trained, it opens up the number of people who are confident and comfortable talking about mental health, and can support colleagues who are struggling. Conversations about mental health are tiring and sometimes awkward, and making yourself vulnerable enough to explain how you are feeling requires bravery. If your school develops a culture of openness and honesty between staff, it will help to limit the shame surrounding mental ill health and help colleagues on their journey to recovery in whatever form that takes.

The first day back to school in September with large meetings, data, folders and being inside all day can be overwhelming and stressful for staff. Showing staff that you are not afraid to try something different to support their mental health takes a brave move from the leadership team of a school. However, staff will immediately recognize that you care about their mental health from the start of the year.

It may be that at the start of the new academic year your school could have a range of staff wellbeing activities instead of the typical rigid meetings schedule. This will create a sense of belonging for new members of staff, allow old friends and colleagues to catch up about their summer holidays, dramas and achievements, and choose an activity to support their wellbeing. There could be a quiet reading corner with wellbeing books, board games, pebble painting, a Nerf gun battle or a game of Rounders. It needs to give everyone the option of picking something that appeals to them and should not be 'forced wellbeing'. Staff will value this as a way to cope with any first day of school anxieties. It is a huge change in routine for people coming back to school after six weeks of lots of self-care, sunshine, socializing, family and all those things that protect our mental health.

There are awful stories on Twitter of schools providing compulsory activities for staff that actually have an adverse effect on some people's mental health. One PE teacher was asked to plan all the first day back compulsory sporting wellbeing activities, which left him feeling anxious and exhausted. Enforced wellbeing is an oxymoron in many ways. People working in schools must be seen as individuals, and some may love choosing their favourite pair of trainers to do a sports activity. For others, insecurities about their physical appearance or health problems may leave them feeling alienated or patronized. After the first school week back, there were a myriad of examples on Twitter where schools completely missed the point when it came to staff wellbeing. One example that summed this up from @conscious schools cited common 'Wellbeing gaffes as: Doughnuts in the staffroom on a Friday, ineffective mindfulness sessions by inexperienced teachers, being required to do yoga or singing on an INSET day, and wellbeing goody bags containing Diet Coke and sweets.' If these things are happening in your schools, it may be an early indication of staff mental health and wellbeing being a mere 'tick box' activity.

Breaks and lunchtimes

- Schedule your staff to do a break duty with a colleague who is a friend.

- They should also be able to do their duty near to their classroom, so that those precious minutes are not wasted commuting to and from their duty.

- Staff should be able to do different things during their lunchtimes. For example, staff who struggle with anxiety may want to have lunch with a trusted colleague in a quiet place to re-charge. Others might like the hustle and bustle of the busy staffroom (even if there is a disturbing lack of cutlery there!). Some might need to go off site to get some fresh air and make a phone call to a loved one.

- It is also important for senior leaders to be present and visible during lunchtimes so that staff can speak to them face-to-face about any concerns they might have. If staff are struggling with their mental health, the security of being able to check in with someone from the leadership team during lunchtimes could be the difference between them coping with the afternoon and needing to leave.

Wellbeing Week

Every year in November, when it is getting cold and darker in the evenings, it may be a good idea for your school to have a staff Wellbeing Week. This must be part of a broader understanding of mental health and be led by people who are considerate of staff wellbeing the whole year round. It might be a good idea to publish this on the official school calendar so that all staff are aware of it. Some ideas could be that there are no after-school meetings or report writing for the week. Staff could opt in to being a wellbeing buddy for the week, which means that they have to look after their wellbeing buddy anonymously by putting gifts in pigeonholes, making cups of tea or other kind treats. It will give a warm glow to staff when they come into school and find something nice in their pigeonhole, and, as Plato famously said, 'caring about the happiness of others, we find our own.'

I cannot overemphasize small acts of kindness that go a long way during a busy teaching day; for example, making a cup of tea for someone who is on break duty, offering to collect paper for the photocopier and generally offering cakes, biscuits or fruit on your birthday to share with colleagues. Our data manager makes THE best cakes in the world, and she baked a homemade Victoria sponge with fresh cream and strawberries. On a Friday when I was feeling tired after a busy week of dealing with Year 11 exam stress, the kind email offering a slice of cake AND the quality of the cake made the rest of the day seem like a breeze.

Family commitments and events

Teaching staff often work long hours and have numerous after-school events such as parents' evenings, which means that they will miss out on all-important family time. Juggling a busy family life comes as part of the demands of teaching, but these exceptional events should be considered as reasonable for staff to be able to ask to have time off to attend them. It could mean that staff offer to cover for each other during these times to avoid expensive cover teachers being involved.

Possible family commitments and events:

- child's first day at school sessions
- child's nativity play (who doesn't want to see their child dressed as an angel singing 'Away in a Manger'?)
- child's sports day
- child's special awards event
- immediate family wedding (many non-teaching people in the 'real world' choose to get married during the week, as it's much cheaper)
- family graduations
- family funerals
- when staff are moving house (one of the most stressful events

in people's lives) they could be given a 'moving day' to help cope with the stress

- attending medical appointments for family members staff are carers for (including children).

Encouraging work–life balance

According to Education Support's *Teacher Wellbeing Index 2019*, 74 per cent of educational professionals stated that they found it hard to switch off from work, which could lead to them neglecting self-care and having positive relationships with friends and family. Factors that led to a poor work–life balance were working long hours on weekdays, not having enough time to be with family and friends, working over the weekend and working over the holidays.

It can be very easy for teachers to take emotional baggage and stress home from the job because school staff genuinely care about the children in their school, and if they have disclosed a traumatic and upsetting event, it can be hard to let that go and enjoy an evening out with friends or family.

Leaders in schools have a responsibility to encourage a good work–life balance among school staff, and they can do this in a variety of ways. They are role models for younger and less-experienced teachers, and it is important that they share their hobbies and interests outside of school; for example, going to the cinema, taking their children to a special event, running charity races, a book they've read or an instrument they play. It is important for senior leaders to show that they have a life outside of school and that they are human beings too. Among leadership teams in schools, where there can be lots of pressure and accountability, the conversations people remember with other leaders are about holidays, getting a new dog and other important life events, not the hours of meetings and policies they sat through together. Having a genuine interest in the lives of the people they line manage is important. This is not being nosey and prying into people's personal lives; letting staff know that it is okay to spend time planning social activities or physical activities that are good for mental health is important. If leaders are perceived as robots that have no life outside of school, this is not good for staff as they will not normalize a good work–life balance, which can then lead to poor mental health.

Case study: #teacher5aday

Some schools have Monday morning whole-staff briefings; some of these could focus on staff self-care suggestions and ideas. I was lucky enough to go to a Twilight Teacher's wellbeing session at Chichester Cathedral and met Naomi Ward, who was an English teacher but who now runs various different training sessions and is a coach. The session was called #teacher5aday and went through the five key areas that staff need to focus on for their own mental health and wellbeing. We were given a copy of her *#teacher5aday Journal and Handbook* (Ward 2014) which goes through reflective exercises to allow busy school staff to stop and think about their lives in a positive and mindful manner. The five areas she suggests are important to prioritize for wellbeing are: connecting, learning, noticing, volunteering and exercising. There is a Twitter support community for teachers to share successes with each other and be part of a group of like-minded professionals who wish to improve their self-care. These are not things to do just as a response to poor mental health, but are important to include in your routine regularly to protect yourself from the risk factors that lead to mental ill health.

The first of the five things that teachers should do is *connecting* with others. This could be by phoning someone for a chat to see how they are instead of texting, spending time reconnecting with a relative you have been meaning to call for months, or asking someone how they are and listening intently and giving them the time and space to talk. The psychological and physical benefits of connecting with someone authentically are huge. Your body will release more endorphins and give your brain 'happy chemicals' that can repair and combat any cortisol that has been released through stress.

The second part is *learning*. This could be any range of things, from learning a new recipe, a new instrument, how to sing, a new language or some other skill that requires spending time dedicated to self-improvement in a way that interests you. It also engages your brain in a way that will combat stress and gives your self-esteem a boost, which may be needed after a tiring day.

The third part is about *noticing* things. We go through our lives absorbed in technology and sometimes forget to go outside and notice the beauty of nature. Noticing things is also about being grateful for things in your life and noticing and being mindful of your feelings. Our lifestyles today are so busy that our brains can get overloaded and overstimulated, which means we neglect the simple things that can improve our mental health and general sense of wellbeing. There is a whole range of mindfulness books and courses available alongside apps such a Headspace and Calm that have guided recordings to aid focusing on the present moment. Many professional sports teams and even members of the Houses of Parliament have been trained on the benefits of living in the moment rather than regretting the past or worrying about the future. The app Calm is free for educators, which helps teachers to practise the skills before possibly using them in their lessons.

The fourth part is *volunteering*. When I heard this I immediately thought, all school staff do is volunteer for things on a daily basis – helping out a distressed child during their morning break, offering to run a school trip, and any other random situation when a colleague pops into your class to ask a 'favour'. However, it could be that staff have other talents they could volunteer. For example, next year I am hoping to volunteer at a great charity called The Wave Project that helps children with special needs learn how to surf. Other friends I know volunteer to raise money for charities by doing different sponsored sporting events. It has to be something you feel passionate about and that will allow you to feel that you are giving back in some way. It cannot be something that is draining and eventually leads to resentment. The problem with working in a school environment is that it takes so much of you that you might feel too tired to find the time to volunteer. And that's fine if you have people depending on your time outside of school. It could be an opportunity to do something you love with like-minded people and you feel like an individual, not just a 'teacher'.

The fifth part is *exercising*. I have asthma, so there are times of the year when I find it hard to exercise outside – usually when it is too hot or too cold. However, I know how important it is to my mental health. Our school has a gym with a swimming pool a 5-minute walk away. They offer a corporate discount to staff for them to use the facilities there. When it is dark outside it is nice to go into the warmth of the gym or pool and to start the day with some serotonin-producing exercise. It genuinely sets me up for the day and makes me feel good that I've spent some time on myself. Other colleagues I know prefer to go at the end of the day; however, a word of warning – there are usually things related to the school day or a meeting after school that can get in the way of your session, so you will need to be flexible. Two of my colleagues started Park Run as a way to look after their mental health. It's an excellent idea as it's free and local, and is a manageable distance of 5km. One of my colleagues is a trained yoga instructor so does this regularly, and others enjoy a long run on a Sunday morning. Another colleague who hadn't exercised for years started playing badminton with her husband on Tuesday evenings. Ultimately, exercise doesn't have to be something that is expensive, but it can make a huge overall difference in your mental health if it is a regular part of your routine. One of my colleagues takes their dog for an extra walk in the evenings for some vital headspace.

After reading Naomi's book you could create a 10-minute Monday morning staff wellbeing briefing session to give them a summary of the #teacher5aday, and ask them to write a pledge to themselves to promise to start prioritizing their mental health. They could select one of the five strands to try to fit into their weekly routine.

Maslow's esteem needs

Valuing staff

Higher up on Maslow's hierarchy of needs is a sense of being valued. Staff in a busy school environment should feel valued as individuals in order to mentally cope with the demands of the job. Many good teachers are being forced out of the profession through schools not investing in their staff, even if it doesn't cost any money.

If staff have had a learning walk or lesson observation by a senior leader or other visitor to the school, they should receive positive feedback via email by the evening of the same day. This means the member of staff feels valued and is not left to worry about the outcome of the visit overnight or longer. There could be two positive comments and one suggestion for improvement that is a supportive and developmental statement. If they have had extra stress and pressure by having a visitor in their classroom, it is only right to congratulate them on their successes as soon as possible.

Year 11 teachers who hold extra revision sessions at weekends or holidays could receive a 'golden ticket' to have an afternoon or morning off in lieu during the summer term. This is a lovely treat and shows how valued teachers are. It allows them to plan an extra family event or birthday treat with loved ones and makes a huge difference. Teachers often hold extra sessions out of the kindness of their hearts and do not expect anything in return. The fact that this kindness is being repaid goes a long way to boost staff mental health. They could go to the cinema with their loved one when it is quiet one afternoon, and it gives them special time away from work to treat themselves. This doesn't cost the school any money as most staff will take it when they have their 'gained time' from when their exam classes have left. In other schools, some members of the senior leadership team offer to cover them when possible.

Acknowledging staff

Schools rely on staff working beyond their allocated hours and they can continue to do this in a manageable way as long as they feel acknowledged for their efforts. The sheer logistics of organizing an extra school trip before you even go can take hours and hours. Many extra events such as the Duke of Edinburgh Award can even take away valuable self-care weekends.

Staff could be acknowledged in the following ways:

- Organize a regular opportunity to thank staff each week publicly (even if people find it embarrassing – if it is done regularly and sincerely, it really supports staff happiness).

- The headteacher and other staff could write personal thank you cards to staff for particular events that they have run. This costs very little, but is valued by staff, and they often display them in their classrooms as a nice reminder whilst they are marking folders and books.

- When staff have weddings or civil partnerships, babies, sporting successes or a promotion, this could be acknowledged in morning staff briefings.

Maslow's self-actualization needs

Happy school staff have various opportunities for growth, either within their current school or alongside their current role. This means that they have conversations that help them to fulfil their potential, professionally and personally. They may wish to complete a Master's, but they just need the extra push from someone at school who believes in them. They may need to reduce their hours to spend time caring for their parents. They may want to study an evening course, but are worried they will be judged by some staff as not being committed. In order for staff to be self-actualized, they must be able to discuss their hopes and dreams for the future with colleagues who genuinely care and want to support them to achieve this. Schools need to have structures in place to have these conversations with staff, and it will lead to happier schools with the potential for staff to flourish and to be the best teachers they can be. They should not be made to feel guilty if they want to pursue opportunities outside of education alongside their teaching career. If this happens in schools, good teachers are likely to leave the profession entirely as it can be made to feel like the system is too inflexible to be a part of.

Rogers' counselling skills and what they look like in a school setting

I am not suggesting that teachers become counsellors for their colleagues, as they do not always have the time or supervision structures in place to keep them safe. What Rogers' work can be used for within a school setting is to provide a framework of skills that staff can learn in order to become more supportive colleagues to those who are struggling with mental ill health. The skills that Carl Rogers developed in order for his clients to reach the state of happiness through self-actualization can be used and kept in mind during a conversation about mental health within a school environment.

Rogers' first skill of *unconditional positive regard* means that the person who is listening to a distressed colleague needs to accept and support them irrespective of what they say. As Rogers says,

> ...when the therapist is experiencing a positive, acceptant attitude toward whatever the client is at that moment, therapeutic movement or change is more likely to occur. The therapist is willing for the client to be whatever immediate feeling is going on – confusion, resentment, fear, anger, courage, love, or pride. Such caring on the part of the therapist is non-possessive. The therapist prizes the client in a total rather than a conditional way. (Rogers 1980, p.116)

If a colleague is struggling with their mental health they will need to be listened to in a way that encourages self-reflection and gives them the time and space to be heard. This will leave them feeling genuinely cared for and will help their path to recovery with signposting to resources that could be helpful.

An example of unconditional positive regard could be something like the following:

> A colleague who is regularly looking tearful and upset comes to talk to you complaining about workload and has been struggling to meet deadlines. You notice that they have been losing weight and have been looking more dishevelled. You realize that something bigger than the complaint about workload is going on. They have come up with a completely irrational conspiracy theory about how other people are working less than them and that others get to spend more time with family and friends. The skill of listening with unconditional positive regard must be used in order to sit with their distress and allow them to self-reflect and unpick the root cause of their concerns. If you dismiss their ideas immediately, irrespective of their legitimacy, you could risk them being absent as a result of stress or feeling unheard and uncared for.

Rogers describes the second skill of *empathy* as, 'This kind of sensitive, active listening is exceedingly rare in our lives. We think we listen, but very rarely do we listen with real understanding, true empathy. Yet listening, of this very special kind, is one of the most potent forces for change that I know' (1980, p.116). When people are listening to distressed colleagues it is important not to necessarily give advice in the same way that you would in an everyday conversation. The colleague who is struggling may feel patronized and misunderstood if this happens. The best thing that can happen is that the active listening strategies outlined previously are used in a way that enables the person struggling to feel understood and not ashamed. Brené Brown has an amazing video clip summarizing the difference between empathy and sympathy.[1]

No one wants to talk to an automaton about their uncomfortable feelings if they think they could be lied to or manipulated. Rogers' skill of empathy is a tricky one to train staff on using, as people are either genuine and authentic or they are not. It is more a quality that people have, and when someone is feeling vulnerable and upset due to their poor mental health, they need to know there is someone they can trust within the school environment. This will usually be based on how open and vulnerable the person is prepared to be with others. The colleague who is listening to a distressed team member should show a warm and human approach that uses body language suggesting they have the time and space to REALLY listen. It is perfectly acceptable when someone talks about their mental health issues to say something along the lines of, 'I am not sure what to say but I am really grateful that you have shared it with me.' This will hopefully build their self-esteem as they begin to feel more confident 'owning their story'. There should be a wide range of people in school who are trained on having supportive conversations about mental health with colleagues because they are choosing to, rather than because it is a compulsory requirement.

1 See www.youtube.com/watch?v=1Evwgu369Jw

CHAPTER 4

Preventative Measures

How to Change Your School Environment to Support Positive Mental Health

Workload

Many teachers can show signs of poor mental health when their workload is particularly high. This usually happens when the marking is adding up, the hours of sunlight each day are getting shorter, they have reports to write or a parents' evening to attend. Signs of this may be shouting at the photocopier that has just eaten their worksheet or, worse, snapping at other members of staff or students. It can be easy to silently judge behaviour like this, but actually, the pressure of an increased workload can really take its toll on mental health in school staff. The guilt that teachers feel when they go for a swim instead of re-planning a lesson can be immense, which can easily become a dangerous cycle of feeling guilty, neglecting self-care routines, suffering from anxiety or depression, and then not being able to focus or work at all.

Funding issues within schools mean that teaching staff have less PPA (planning, preparation and assessment) time than before, so they inevitably have to do more work before or after school, at weekends or in the holidays. The Department for Education completed a Teacher Workload Survey in 2019. This was a month-long survey where 20,704 school teachers, middle leaders and senior leaders responded to suggest ways that schools could reduce unnecessary workload. The three main areas that teachers said were unnecessary were: the amount of marking they were required to do, the amount of lessons they had to plan and the management of data that was required.

In the more recent *Teacher Wellbeing Index 2019*, 71 per cent of educational professionals surveyed cited workload as the contributing factor towards them wanting to leave the profession. Teaching is often seen as a vocation rather than as a profession, and there is no physical way that a full-time secondary school teacher could fit their workload into the 32.5 hours a week they are paid for – 33 per cent of teachers work more than 51 hours a week (Education Support 2019). There is a clear link between the number of hours worked and the level of impact this has on mental health. This means that, up to a tipping point, teachers expect to work in the evenings and at weekends to prepare lessons, mark student work and do any other administration tasks such as writing reports. However, if this is not well planned by the leadership team, well publicised and staff are not supported by someone, all this workload can feel overwhelming. If it is constant and making the body release the stress hormone cortisol, staff will get 'burned out' mentally or become physically unwell and be unable to teach.

The Ofsted *Teacher Well-being* report (2019a, p.6) found that 'the main causes of heavy workload are: the volume of administrative tasks, the volume of marking, staff shortages, lack of support from external agencies, challenging behaviour of students, changes to external examinations, frequently changing UK Government policies and regulations, and in some cases lack of skills or training.' In this chapter I will look at these to suggest ideas to support staff mental health.

There are some cheap practical steps that schools can take to manage workload effectively, starting with the organization of the school staff calendar. When the calendar is compiled at any school there are steps that the leadership team can take to ensure that it is well balanced. For example, they could ensure that there is never an after-school meeting in a week when there is a parents' evening. There could be clear and manageable time periods for report writing and any centralized or end of year exams. The data capture points and after-school meetings could be scheduled to allow staff to organize family commitments and self-care around them. The annual calendar could be available to staff before they break up for the summer so that they have plenty of warning about events in the new academic year. If this is not happening in your school, you might want to tactfully ask why this is the case. Staff need to be able to organize and manage their workload to help them feel on top of things and relieve anxieties about not being able to 'stay afloat'.

Senior leadership teams should evaluate any changes that add to staff workload and be prepared to respond to staff feedback. Being honest with staff about recognizing workload changes is important, and sharing the bigger picture with staff often helps to contextualize the reasons for the changes. In July 2018, the UK Government introduced the *School Workload Reduction Toolkit* that contains resources to identify, address and evaluate workload issues in schools. Senior and middle leaders could use this to evaluate the impact of any new initiatives on staff workload and wellbeing (DfE 2018).

Marking policy

All the research demonstrates how important feedback is to students in terms of them developing their learning and making good progress, but it has to be meaningful and manageable for staff. It can be so rewarding to see how students who have struggled grasping an idea show how they have progressed during the lessons you have taught them. We all know the time that marking takes, particularly for teachers of essay-based subjects. In schools up and down the country, English teachers during mock exam periods are often seen with wheelie suitcases full of papers and a soulless look behind the eyes. The hours that teachers can spend marking can be tiring and draining, and may prevent staff ensuring that they are protecting their mental health. I know at the end of a busy day that staff may need to watch a familiar film or have a swim and not have to read reams of paper. If there is a clear marking policy, staff are able to carefully plan their marking schedule and it feels more manageable and meaningful. You don't want to hear about staff neglecting their families or not being able to go their exercise class because they had a pile of assessments or tests to mark. Nor should it be an expectation that this happens.

Ideally, marking policies should be developed in consultation with staff and take into account the number of lessons each subject has, to ensure equity. There should be no need to 'tick and flick' every page of a folder or workbook. All subjects are expected to mark one piece of work for every set quantity of teaching, for example every eight hours. This could be marked giving one 'improvement step' and a chance for students to respond to this to improve their work during the follow-up lesson's 'reflection time'. Self-assessment and peer assessment could be regularly used in lessons to minimize staff marking. Spelling mistakes need to be corrected in line with a policy, for example for the first three spellings only. If there is a consistent and standardized approach to marking, it gives a familiar experience for all students, and allows staff to manage their workload. Additionally, it potentially allows students to value the time that has been spent marking by using that feedback to improve their response during 'reflection time'. This is very important as for teachers who regularly mark long essays, any potential resentment they may have will be quickly washed away by seeing the students respond well to the feedback, happy that students can then improve their work and recognize how well they have done.

Lesson planning

Lesson planning is essential to ensure that students are receiving the best possible teaching to make good progress. Good lessons don't happen by chance, and must be carefully considered. I suspect teachers all remember the dark days of their training year where they had to complete minute-by-minute lesson plans which took about 30 minutes to write for every hour lesson they planned. At the time it may have been helpful to learn the process and rehearse the lessons in advance on paper, but the thought of having to do this every day would be enough for many teachers to want to hang up their hats.

The 2014 Department for Education Teacher Workload Survey found that teachers across primary and secondary schools are being asked to complete vast amounts of planning. One example from the Survey found: 'Weekly planning with learning objectives and success criteria for every area of submission to the head of year, due in every Saturday by 5pm. Feedback is given on a Sunday evening with suggestions for "even better if" steps to adapt the lessons.

This takes all day on a Saturday so I have no weekend. I find it demoralizing and soul destroying that my class is outstanding and yet this gives the impression of a lack of trust.'

Having this sort of workload is unsustainable and the constant monitoring can lead people to feel undermined and not trusted. This may start to corrode self-esteem and this level of work can quickly lead to neglecting self-care and people's mental health can start to deteriorate. According to Ofsted's *School Inspection Handbook* (2019b), there is no requirement for teachers to produce lesson plans during an inspection, so schools should seriously consider the justification for asking staff to complete them. Senior leaders need to ask if their staff can use their time in a more meaningful way that gives them time to look after their mental health, and will therefore make them better teachers.

Another aspect to this that was noted in Ofsted's *Teacher Well-being* report (2019a) is that more teachers are being expected to teach a second subject. This may be due to a need within the timetable and the fact that they have completed the subject at GCSE themselves a number of years ago. However, this added pressure without adequate time for planning can cause added stress and a constant state of fear that they will not know the answer to a random question on the subject from an especially inquisitive student. It can be an extremely stressful time as the lessons may need adapting but teachers may not have the knowledge or the resources to do this. More experienced colleagues may be able to support their colleagues, and *Tes* provides some excellent free resources. Schools could also host 'subject network hub meetings' with other local schools that are part of their academy chain. This is a good opportunity to complete some collaborative planning with a team of staff with various backgrounds and experience. Having scheduled time once every half-term working with teaching teams to plan new resources and work together could help to ease the anxiety.

Parents' evenings

Parents' evenings can be a lovely opportunity to meet parents to give face-to-face praise and feedback on their children. They can also be the time to share honest truths about how things need to change, which can be stressful. In secondary schools, some teachers may have to attend up to seven different parents' evenings throughout the academic year. After a busy school day, when teachers want to go home, change into their pyjamas and watch a box set on Netflix, they have to spend at least another three hours talking to a range of parents who require their undivided attention. Parents' evenings can cause a lot of anxiety among staff and some extra staff TLC goes a long way.

Tips to support staff wellbeing at parents' evenings:

- Online booking systems: these save teachers' time, and can automatically pre-book 15-minute breaks for teachers to get fresh air, use the bathroom and stretch their legs.

- School finishing early for students: having this time out gives staff some space to recharge from the mental strain of conversations, and allows them time to get extra food to fuel their brains, if needed. Having this downtime is essential for staff to feel human instead of feeling like automatons. Teaching for a whole day with all its challenges is mentally tiring in itself, but to expect staff to carry on through until 7pm without breathing space is not good for their mental health.

- Scheduling parents' evenings on a Thursday night: this means tired staff will only have to get through one day of teaching before the weekend to recharge.
- The senior leadership team should be popping round to make sure everything is going well, having a supportive chat and making their presence known. This enables staff to feel that they can redirect any unreasonable or irate parents if needed (luckily these are very rare), and they feel supported and cared for by the leadership team.
- Consider the location for parents' evenings. A loud busy room could mean that teachers have to strain their voices to be heard over other conversations. This could result in staff losing their voices and/or sanity. However, there must be a balance so that parents are not spending time trying to decipher a map of different locations and teachers.

Email protocols

In an environment like schools, when every minute is precious, it is often easier to fire off an email rather than have a conversation, particularly when your school is spread over a large site. The ability to share valuable information that can help support vulnerable children can be so useful. However, this is not always the best way for staff to work, and more stress and workload can be created when someone misunderstands a message and does something that makes life harder.

As the Ofsted *Teacher Well-being* report found:

> Communication between staff and parents represents another issue. An open access to staff email addresses creates an expectation and pressure for an immediate response from staff (including senior leaders and headteachers). Some schools even have a 'culture of competition' in which parents share schools' response rates among themselves. As a result, the instant response email culture adds to workload and interferes with work–life balance: 'My email inbox is like a pit of death. My emails are incessant. I often receive 50–80 emails per day, even when I am ill. Some of these are important, but it means I have to sift through them to make sure I get to the important things.' 'Parents email at night and want an instant response that night. If you don't respond that night, they phone the school the next day.' In view of the workload issues and lack of work–life balance discussed earlier, the 'instant response culture' is not trivial. Steps should be taken to address this problem. (Ofsted 2019a, pp.37–38)

Tips and ideas for email protocols:

- Do not allow school staff members to make the mistake of attaching their work emails to their smartphones.
- Schools may not have an official policy on emails, but no one should be expected to check or write emails 24/7.

- If a parent emails it should be generally expected that they will receive a reply within 48 hours (unless it's a weekend or a holiday).
- School staff should not get mad late-night headteachers' demand emails, as some people have reported from their schools in the past.
- It should not be in a school's culture to send emails late at night and expect things to be done by the following morning.
- During holidays, staff should be able to put an 'out of office' on their emails so that parents can understand when they can expect a reply.
- Avoid a one-size-fits-all policy for email protocols so that staff manage their emails in a way that suits their lifestyle.
- Do not expect staff to reply to emails over the weekend.

Report writing

Writing reports can be a useful way of communicating to parents how their children are progressing. We all know that in schools some teachers will be responsible for a higher number of classes than others. For example, core subject teachers see their students more often and have fewer classes, whereas creative subject teachers will see students less often and have more classes in total. This creates an issue for staff wellbeing during report-writing periods. If they are scheduled into a school's calendar during the year, then staff will know when the deadlines are, and can balance them in their workload. Some schools have reduced the quantity of time needing to be spent by entering an 'attitude to learning' grade from a drop-down menu and a projected grade (what they should achieve at the end of the year) as a progress check twice a year. For the full written reports, staff could be given a guidance document as to the structure, so that it is consistent between subjects. Teachers should be allowed to copy and paste statements, within reason, and there is a word limit. This process means that for some teachers, they will have trickier times of the year and may need support to manage their report writing and self-care.

Other schools have shifted towards not writing long reports, just a report on progress once a term, which is selected from a drop-down menu. Ultimately, parents' evenings are already an opportunity to discuss a child's progress, and, unless something is going drastically wrong, is there a need to have report writing at all in schools? I don't have the answer to this, but prioritizing staff mental health may mean not needing to spend hours copying and pasting comments into a report that may not even be read by parents.

Behaviour policy

Teachers have all had the steep learning curve in their teacher training year when they are given sole control of the class with a range of behaviour issues that they have been having nightmares about for weeks. You spent hours observing their behaviour with a mentor leading the way. You've marked their folders, learned all their names and special educational needs. On a one-to-one basis you have good relationships with them. Then suddenly, when you took the helm, they smelt your fear and started throwing paper at each other and the smallest red-haired boy in the class shouted at you, 'You don't know what you are doing!' To which you realized you really didn't. At this point the choice is to either to go home, have a good cry and share the story in a humorous way in a book about teacher mental health many years later, or you break down and leave the profession. The power of poor behaviour in the classroom can really affect a teacher's mental health and their ability to function. This is why schools need to provide support for staff to help them to feel supported and in control of their learning environment.

According to the *Teacher Well-being Index 2018*, managing student behaviour is the third most important reason for teachers leaving the profession. For staff who had admitted to suffering with symptoms of mental ill health, 43 per cent stated that this was due to having to manage student behaviour. This was an increase of 9 per cent from the last survey in 2017. Whilst staff are expected to manage student behaviour as part of their role, the overall behaviour system needs to be fit for purpose in order to protect staff mental health. According to the Teaching and Learning International Survey (TALIS) (Ainley and Carstens 2018), England's schools ranked 13th out of 48 countries for levels of teacher intimidation. This can lead to poor mental health in staff if not rectified and dealt with by a behaviour system that supports staff.

Teenagers are by their very nature risk-taking. Their limbic systems are still growing in their brains and there are so many variables that can lead to poor behaviour. There is an excellent TED talk about this by Kashfia Rahman that could be used during a staff training session on teenage mental health.[1] There is not a

1 See www.ted.com/talks/kashfia_rahman_how_risk_taking_changes_a_teenager_s_brain?language=en

classroom in the land where students are perfectly compliant and learning every single lesson because teenagers are hormonal, unpredictable and heavily influenced by peer pressure and an all-consuming desire to challenge authority. Therefore, your behaviour system needs to have the capacity and procedures to deal with poor behaviour, when it arises, in a swift way that doesn't add to teacher workload. It also needs to have a restorative component so that the student has an opportunity to repair any damage to the working relationship caused by poor behaviour choices. Staff need to see the system working and be able to go home knowing that the behaviour has been dealt with and that they can switch off from thinking about it for the evening.

Underpinning the watertight system must be reinforcement from the senior leadership team. However, the Ofsted *Teacher Well-being* report (2019a, p.7), found that senior leaders are not always seen as providing sufficient support for managing pupils' behaviour. According to many respondents, senior leaders do not work with teachers when it is necessary to solve discipline problems jointly, and the issues are made worse by an inconsistent approach to managing behaviour.

Lack of senior leadership support with managing poor behaviour is one of the main ways in which senior leaders negatively influence wellbeing in schools and further education and skills (FES) providers. The issue is two-fold. First, there is a lack of support from senior leaders: 'Pupil behaviour – no visible SLT [senior leadership team] support during known "hotspot" times.' 'No behaviour policy.' Only 45 per cent of respondents from FES providers and 56 per cent of respondents from schools report that senior leaders collaborate with teachers when they need to solve classroom discipline problems jointly. Second, there is an inconsistent approach to managing behaviour: 'Behavioural policy that is not followed consistently, even by the people who wrote it... Lack of consistency among staff when dealing with poor behaviour' (Ofsted 2019a, p.36).

This doesn't always have to be the case. In some schools there is a clear system with different sanctions for different behaviour. Ideally, this is all recorded online so that parents can access the information. If a student is set an after-school detention, then the member of staff who has issued it to them could attend the start of the detention to have a restorative conversation with the student about their behaviour and set any work they have missed in the lesson. This is an excellent way to repair the working relationship and ease the anxiety of the next lesson for both the student and staff member. The behaviour policy must be consistently used among all staff members so that they support each other and share the same expectations. The school leadership team have to be brave enough to admit when it might need changing and be clear about the impact it could have on staff in terms of workload and changes to their routine.

In your school, if you are feeling undermined by a behaviour system that doesn't support you, or that is ineffective or outdated, this must change to preserve staff mental health. It should never be the case that a member of staff goes home feeling bullied or upset by a student's behaviour because inevitably this can start to lead to a poor mental health coping strategy such as alcohol, gambling, over-eating or even cause behaviour such as self-harming. There can be systems that support staff managing behaviour, and allow them to feel like they can go to school the next day without suffering from anxiety and worry. It won't stop occasional poor behaviour choices from hormonal teenagers, but it can leave staff feeling empowered and in control of the situation.

Meetings

Meetings after school can be tiring and add extra stress and strain after a busy day teaching. They must be run in a meaningful way in order to protect staff mental health.

Tips and ideas to make meetings meaningful:

- They should be kept to a minimum during peak workload times of the year such as report-writing weeks, mock exam marking and parents' evenings.
- Colleagues who are struggling with their mental health should have the option of not attending big meetings, but make sure that they get a copy of the meeting notes so that they don't feel left out of the loop.
- There should be no more than one after-school meeting or CPD session each week.
- After-school meetings should be no longer than an hour in length as our brains can only take so much information in at the end of a busy working day.
- If you are part of the leadership team creating the meeting schedule in your school, it is important to have a balance of departmental and pastoral meetings.
- Pastoral or year team meetings are useful to talk about specific students and share ideas and strategies.

- Leadership teams need to be prepared to be flexible and adapt to their staff. If you have times in the year when absence is high – typically in the winter months when different illnesses are doing the rounds and people are tired due to a lack of daylight – it may be a good idea to cancel a calendared meeting and let your staff know why.

CHAPTER 5

Activity

Putting the Theory into Practice

Whilst it is useful to learn about mental health theoretically, it is often more helpful to check you have understood the key concepts and examples of best practice by applying them to different scenarios. Four scenarios are presented here, with potential solutions given in Appendix 2.

Scenarios to explore how to support colleagues

Scenario 1

Someone working in your department has been absent from school on a few random days with ailments such as a migraine or upset stomach. They have also asked for a couple of afternoons off to attend unspecified medical appointments. They have become isolated and have been hiding in their classroom at lunchtime instead of joining in with the rest of the faculty. They pop into your office at the end of the day to tell you that they have been put on anti-depressants and have been struggling to function. They have been diagnosed with depression and have been put on a waiting list for counselling sessions.

Which practical steps could you use to restructure their workload and make 'reasonable adjustments' to account for their mental health condition?

____

____

____

____

How could you encourage them to explain what support they might need?

____

____

____

____

Scenario 2

A member of staff has just come back from paternity leave. It is his first baby and he has recently taken a promotion as head of subject to support his family. He is looking tired and has mentioned to other colleagues about how his wife is struggling with PND, is really unhappy and he has been caring for her. He has been absent from various after-school meetings and he is behind with his report-writing deadlines.

Why is he more likely to be at risk of developing mental ill health?

Which questions would be appropriate to ask to make sure he is getting the right support he needs?

How could unconditional positive regard towards him ensure that he feels supported?

Scenario 3

A colleague has been having counselling sessions to help her to cope with the sudden death of her partner. She likes the routine of work and is usually an excellent teacher. She has worked at the school for 23 years and is an excellent role model for the younger teachers. However, she has recently been returning to work after sessions and delivering poor lessons, snapping at other colleagues and complaining about her workload.

Who would be the best person to have a conversation with her about her mental health?

How could empathy be used in the conversation?

____

____

____

____

Which practical steps could be taken to support her?

____

____

____

____

Scenario 4

A colleague has come to you as their headteacher to tell you that he is struggling with an eating disorder that is a symptom of his ongoing anxiety. As a result, he has been over-exercising, eating less and losing weight. He has recently separated from his wife and has been struggling to keep on top of his teaching commitments.

How could you speak to him using congruence?

Where could you signpost him to?

Which practical steps could you put in place to support him?

Conclusion

Working in schools with children can be the most rewarding vocation in the world. I am concluding this book at the start of the school year, and wanted to share some of the 'little gems' of situations I have experienced within my first week back. These will carry me through any teenage strop, tantrum, meltdown or unkindness:

- The sheer delight of a child smiling at me as they come into my classroom for the first time, look at the worksheet task I have given them and say 'These are my favourite – I love these', and then walk away to their seat as if I had just given them £1000.
- The children who finish their work and then instinctively offer to help a friend they can see is struggling with theirs.
- Two Year 7 boys who spontaneously start dancing (in sync) to a video clip we are watching and not feeling self-conscious.

- The chain of 'Thank you for the lesson' at the end as they leave my classroom to rush off to their next lesson.

- The boy whose pen has somehow exploded covering both hands with sticky black ink, desperately trying not to laugh at the ridiculousness of the situation.

- The student who wants to swing by at break time to tell me about the extra revision they have been doing for my subject and wants to share that with me (I listened for 10 minutes then politely told him I needed to make a cup of tea and use the bathroom before my next lesson).

- Two students totally absorbed in writing an acrostic poem and then proudly reading it out to me together, spontaneously.

- A student who smiles at me and tells me this is the best lesson of the day.

- Popping into the library to see some students reading and completely losing themselves in the story.

- A student opening a door for a teacher without being asked.

- Colleagues supporting each other by making cups of tea for others at break time.

- A form group Jenga competition, which was played with utter professionalism.

However, these rose-tinted moments are not the full picture.

If they were, teachers wouldn't be leaving the profession in the numbers they are.

At the end of the first week the slow erosion of the mental health of my colleagues has begun:

- I have seen a teacher in tears because a student she had cared for had been particularly nasty to her in a lesson.
- A burnt-out NQT who hadn't been looking after himself and was tearful and sad as a result.
- Someone who said their week had been 'non-stop' and another who discussed the concept of 'treat wees' – the idea that when you have done some work, you can treat yourself with a visit to the bathroom.
- Another whose first free period of the week wasn't until Friday and was shattered.
- Someone who wouldn't have made herself a cup of coffee as she had no free periods and was on break and lunch duty.
- A teacher who had needed to break their healthy eating routine and have chocolate every day in the evening to cope.
- An English teacher who had only managed to read a page of her new fiction book before collapsing asleep.

Even with a rigid self-care routine, I have had to go to bed earlier than I would like a couple of evenings this week just to get the sleep I need after the business of the school day. Our bodies and minds need lots of recovery time to cope with the demands of working in such a busy and emotionally draining role, and the shock on our systems of having to get back into the school routine should not be underestimated. I have planned my self-care into my schedule as if it is non-negotiable in the same way teaching lessons are. I know there will be times during the year I will find this hard to stick to. However, I also know that with the right support and colleagues and friends looking after me, I will continue to be able to prioritize my mental health and self-care so that I can stay in the profession I truly love.

I hope that this book has given people working in schools some practical steps and ideas to do the same because all children need inspiration, as well as a love of learning and kindness in their lives.

APPENDIX 1

Staff Mental Health Survey Questions

1. How would you rate your knowledge of mental ill health?

   Excellent

   Good

   Average

   Poor

2. Are you comfortable talking about your mental health?

   Very comfortable

   Comfortable

Not comfortable

Totally awkward

3. Have you ever experienced mental ill health?

Yes

No

Not sure

4. If you have a mental health diagnosis, which category would it fall into?

Depression

Anxiety

Eating disorder

Psychosis (bi-polar or schizophrenia)

5. If you have absence from work due to mental ill health, have you stated this as the reason for absence and discussed this with your line manager on your return to work?

Yes

No (please explain why below)

N/A

6. Have you ever engaged in talking therapies or taken medication to assist you with your mental health?

Talking therapies

Medication

Both

N/A

7. Would you know how to support a colleague who was suffering from mental ill health?

Yes

No

8. Do you know where you can get help and support within school if you think you might be struggling with mental ill health?

Yes

No

APPENDIX 2

Potential Solutions to Scenarios

Scenario 1

Someone working in your department has been absent from school on a few random days with ailments such as a migraine or upset stomach. They have also asked for a couple of afternoons off to attend unspecified medical appointments. They have become isolated and have been hiding in their classroom at lunchtime instead of joining in with the rest of the faculty. They pop into your office at the end of the day to tell you that they have been put on anti-depressants and have been struggling to function. They have been diagnosed with depression and have been put on a waiting list for counselling sessions.

Which practical steps could you use to restructure their workload and make 'reasonable adjustments' to account for their mental health condition?

- They may need to reduce their hours temporarily to support any side effects of the medication they are starting.
- They may need time off school to attend counselling appointments.
- They may need weekly check-in meetings and support from someone they trust in school.
- You could create a support plan with them to ensure that they can reflect on things that can support their recovery from this period of mental ill health.
- They may need time off school to attend GP appointments to review their medication.

How could you encourage them to explain what support they might need?

- Talking through the support they are entitled to because of the Equality Act and the 'reasonable adjustments' that could be made to support them.
- Signposting them to support services such as the Education Support partnership or other local counselling providers.

Scenario 2

A member of staff has just come back from paternity leave. It is his first baby and he has recently taken a promotion as head of subject to support his family. He is looking tired and has mentioned to other colleagues about how his wife is struggling with PND, is really unhappy and he has been caring for her. He has been absent from various after-school meetings and he is behind with his report-writing deadlines.

Why is he more likely to be at risk of developing mental ill health?

- Carers are more likely to struggle to find the time to complete vital self-care and, as a result, they are much more likely to suffer from mental ill health. He also has certain rights as a carer such as 'reasonable adjustments' to his work.

Which questions would be appropriate to ask to make sure he is getting the right support he needs?

- 'How are you managing the changes of your new family life?'
- 'How much are you having to care for your wife?'
- 'Is there any support that you think we can offer you in school?'
- 'Are there any times when flexible working could be used to help you?'

How could unconditional positive regard towards him ensure that he feels supported?

- He will need to be treated with respect, kindness and given a chance to talk about his worries without being patronized. He will need to be given adequate time that is undisturbed and private.
- Do not give advice to him and do not underestimate the emotional toll that caring can take on a person.

Scenario 3

A colleague has been having counselling sessions to help her to cope with the sudden death of her partner. She likes the routine of work and is usually an excellent teacher. She has worked at the school for 23 years and is an inspiring role model for the younger teachers. However, she has recently been returning to work after sessions and delivering poor lessons, snapping at other colleagues and complaining about her workload.

Who would be the best person to have a conversation with her about her mental health?

- Someone who has worked with her for a number of years and who she trusts and connects with. (This is not necessarily her line manager.)

How could empathy be used in the conversation?

- Using active listening, the person having the conversation will need to listen without interrupting and clarify points to check any misunderstandings.
- They will need to make sure they have spent time asking about specific things that help the colleague to understand how it feels to be in distress about losing a partner.

Which practical steps could be taken to support her?

- Allow her time to recover after counselling sessions to go home and process things, rather than coming straight back into school.
- Set up regular check-in meetings when needed to discuss any changing support needs.

Scenario 4

A colleague has come to you as their headteacher to tell you that he is struggling with an eating disorder that is a symptom of his ongoing anxiety. As a result, he has been over-exercising, eating less and losing weight. He has recently separated from his wife and has been struggling to keep on top of his teaching commitments.

How could you speak to him using congruence?

- Using active listening techniques to convey that you really care about them and are responding with empathy instead of sympathy.

Where could you signpost him to?

- His doctor.

- The Education Support partnership phone line (Tel: 08000 562 561).

- Male eating disorder charities.

Which practical steps could you put in place to support him?

- Offer regular check-ins to ensure that he can discuss his support needs.

- Allow time off for any GP or counselling appointments.

- Ensure he has a plan for exercise each week that can ensure that he has enough time for his teaching commitments.

References

Ainley, J. and Carstens, R. (2018) *Teaching and Learning International Survey (TALIS)*. Paris: Organisation for Economic Co-operation and Development (OECD).

Angelou, M. (1984 [1969]) *I Know Why The Caged Bird Sings*. London: Virago.

Belgutay, J. (2019) 'Meet the mental health advisory panel for teachers.' *Tes*, 5 July. Available at www.tes.com/news/meet-mental-health-advisory-panel-teachers

Brown, B. (2012) *Daring Greatly: How the Courage to Be Vulnerable Transforms the Way We Live, Love, Parent and Lead*. USA: Gotham Books.

Brown, E. (2013) 'Rest and Self-Care are So Important. When You Take Time to Replenish Your Spirit, it Allows You to Serve Others from the Overflow. You Cannot Serve From an Empty Vessell.' *My Spiritual Sabbatical by Eleanor Brownn*. Available at https://eleanorbrownn.wordpress.com/2013/09/04/rest-and-self-care-are-so-important-when-you-take-time-to-replenish-your-spirit-it-allows-you-to-serve-others-from-the-overflow-you-cannot-serve-from-an-empty-vessel

Carers UK (2015) *State of Caring 2015*. London: Carers UK. Available at www.carersuk.org/for-professionals/policy/policy-library/state-of-caring-2015

Cowley, A. (2019) *The Wellbeing Toolkit: Sustaining, Supporting and Enabling School Staff*. London: Bloomsbury Education.

DfE (Department for Education) (2018) *School Workload Reduction Toolkit*. Available at www.gov.uk/guidance/school-workload-reduction-toolkit

DH (Department of Health) (2014) 'The relationship between wellbeing and health.' A Compendium of Factsheets: Wellbeing Across the Lifecourse. Available at https://assets.publishing.service.gov.uk/government/uploads/system/uploads/attachment_data/file/295474/The_relationship_between_wellbeing_and_health.pdf

Downing, N. (2019) 'Wellbeing: Why don't schools offer staff supervision?' *Tes*, 27 June. Available at www.tes.com/news/mental-health-schools-supervision-teachers

Education Business (no date) 'The long and short of the UK teacher crisis.' Available at https://educationbusinessuk.net/features/long-and-short-%c2%a0-uk-teacher-crisis

Education Support (2018) *Teacher Wellbeing Index 2018*. Available at www.education-support.org.uk/resources/research-reports/teacher-wellbeing-index-2018

Education Support (2019) *Teacher Wellbeing Index 2019*. Available at www.education-support.org.uk/sites/default/files/teacher_wellbeing_index_2019.pdf

HSE (Health and Safety Executive) (2018) 'Health and safety statistics.' Available at www.hse.gov.uk/statistics

Kell, E. (2018) *How to Survive in Teaching: Without Imploding, Exploding or Walking Away*. London: Bloomsbury Education.

Maslow, A. (2013 [1943]) *A Theory of Human Motivation*. Radford, VA: Wilder Publications.

Mental Health Foundation (no date) *Managing Mental Health in the Workplace*. London: Mental Health Foundation. Available at www.mentalhealth.org.uk/publications/managing-mental-health-workplace

Mind (no date, a) 'Types of mental health problems.' Available at www.mind.org.uk/information-support/types-of-mental-health-problems

Mind (no date, b) 'Anxiety and panic attacks.' Available at www.mind.org.uk/information-support/types-of-mental-health-problems/anxiety-and-panic-attacks/anxiety-symptoms

Mind (no date, c) 'Obsessive-compulsive disorder (OCD).' Available at www.mind.org.uk/information-support/types-of-mental-health-problems/obsessive-compulsive-disorder-ocd

NAHT (National Association of Headteachers) (2015) 'Recruitment survey shows growing problems in schools.' December. Available at https://www.schoolsweek.co.uk/wp-content/uploads/2015/12/NAHT-recruitment-survey-2015.pdf

NHS (no date, a) 'Symptoms: clinical depression.' Available at www.nhs.uk/conditions/clinical-depression/symptoms

NHS (no date, b) 'Causes: Post-traumatic stress disorder (PTSD).' Available at www.nhs.uk/conditions/post-traumatic-stress-disorder-ptsd/causes

NHS (no date, c) 'Overview: Post-traumatic stress disorder (PTSD).' Available at https://www.nhs.uk/conditions/post-traumatic-stress-disorder-ptsd

NHS Benchmarking Network (2018) '2018 CAMHS Project – Results published.' Available at www.nhsbenchmarking.nhs.uk/news/2018-camhs-project-results-published

Ofsted (2019a) *Teacher Well-being at Work in Schools and Further Education Providers*. Available at www.gov.uk/government/publications/teacher-well-being-at-work-in-schools-and-further-education-providers

Ofsted (2019b) *School Inspection Handbook*. Available at www.gov.uk/government/publications/school-inspection-handbook-eif

ONS (Office for National Statistics (2014) 'Sickness absence in the UK labour market, including number of days lost and reasons for absence.' Available at www.ons.gov.uk/employmentandlabourmarket/peopleinwork/labourproductivity/articles/sicknessabsenceinthelabourmarket/2014-02-25

Pocha, S. K. (2016) 'J.K. Rowling offers touching advice to a fan sufferering depression.' *Stylist*. Available at www.stylist.co.uk/people/j-k-rowling-gives-touching-advice-to-a-fan-suffering-depression-anxiety/27011

Rogers, C. R. (1980) *A Way of Being*. Boston, MA: Houghton-Mifflin.

Sinek, S. 2011) *Start with Why*. London: Penguin.

Speck, D. (2019a) '"Steep rise" in teachers struggling with mental health.' *Tes*, 16 May. Available at www.tes.com/news/steep-rise-teachers-struggling-mental-health

Speck, D. (2019b) 'Mental health "crisis" for trainee teachers.' *Tes*, 16 July. Available at www.tes.com/news/exclusive-mental-health-crisis-trainee-teachers

van der Volk, B. (2015) *The Body Keeps the Score: Mind, Brain, and Body in the Transformation of Trauma*. London: Penguin.

Walker, M., Worth, J. and Van den Brande, J.: National Foundation for Educational Research (2019) 'Teacher Workload Survey 2019. Research Report.' Available at https://assets.publishing.service.gov.uk/government/uploads/system/uploads/attachment_data/file/855933/teacher_workload_survey_2019_main_report_amended.pdf

Ward, N. (ed.) (2014) *#teacher5aday Journal and Handbook*.

WHO (World Health Organization) (2019) 'Mental health.' Available at www.who.int/features/factfiles/mental_health/en

Video clips

Brené Brown (June 2010) 'The power of vulnerability.' TEDxHouston. Available at www.ted.com/talks/brene_brown_the_power_of_vulnerability

Brené Brown (16 March 2012) 'Listening to shame.' TED talk. Available at www.youtube.com/watch?v=psN1DORYYV0

Dr Pooky Knightsmith (5 December 2017) 'Preparing to visit the GP about your mental health.' Available at www.youtube.com/watch?v=PaR-c-tQPTs

Mind (7 June 2016) 'Find the words, How to talk to your GP about your mental health'. Available at www.youtube.com/watch?v=Dqb-n_L5hIA&feature=youtu.be

6 Tips for Active Listening (4 October 2015) Available at www.youtube.com/watch?v=oWe_ogA5YCU

About the Author

Amy Sayer has been a secondary school teacher for the past 13 years. She has completed her NPQSL qualification on supporting disadvantaged students in her school. She is a trained Mental Health First Aider and has previously been her school's mental health and wellbeing lead, helping them to achieve the prestigious Carnegie Centre of Excellence in Mental Health Award in 2019. She has led a roundtable discussion at the Annual Mental Health Conference run by Leeds Beckett University.

Amy has recently had articles published in *Teach Secondary*, *SecEd* and *Tes*. These have been of a range of issues from supporting student mental health, discussions about staff mental health and supporting students with Asperger's Syndrome.

She lives with her husband in Shoreham-by-Sea and loves kayaking, paddleboarding and skateboarding when she is not writing, reading or teaching.

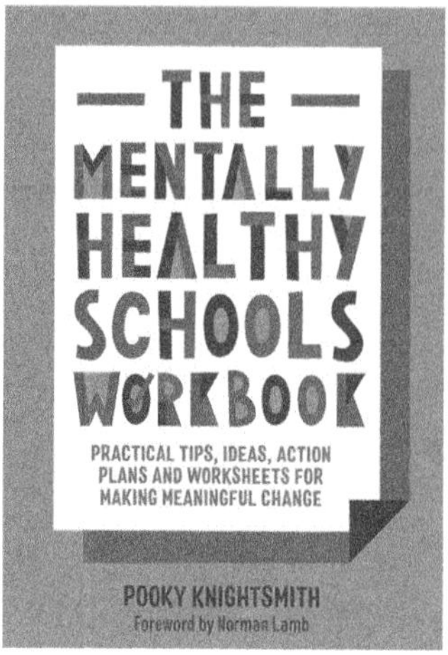

The Mentally Healthy Schools Workbook
Practical Tips, Ideas, Action Plans and Worksheets for Making Meaningful Change
Pooky Knightsmith

Paperback: £19.99/$27.95
ISBN: 978 1 78775 148 4
eISBN: 978 1 78775 149 1
200 pages

This book is the perfect starting point for anyone looking to promote and encourage mental health in their school, or evaluate their existing provision, in line with current government priorities. It covers not only the day-to-day practical steps you can take to meet the mental health needs of learners, but also a provides a whole bank of ideas for ensuring you adopt a whole-school approach to positive mental health.

Pooky Knightsmith lays out tried and tested tools you can use to evaluate the overall mental health of a school, showing how to improve and support the mental health of staff, and how to ensure that the voice of every learner is heard and valued, including the most vulnerable - and that everyone involved with the school feels safe, healthy and happy. Pooky's simple 'litmus test' framework lays out six practical areas you can explore to implement change within your own school, with explanations, sheets to fill in, tips from loads of school staff, and case examples that break these ideas down into easily digestible chunks. This much-needed book is a jumping off point for meaningful change in all aspects of your school community that will promote, support and strengthen mental health at whole-school level.

Pooky Knightsmith has a PhD in child mental health from the Institute of Psychiatry, is the author of five books and is the current vice chair of the Children and Young People's Mental Health Coalition. She has a YouTube channel which is a source of Continuing Professional Development for many educators in the UK and beyond.

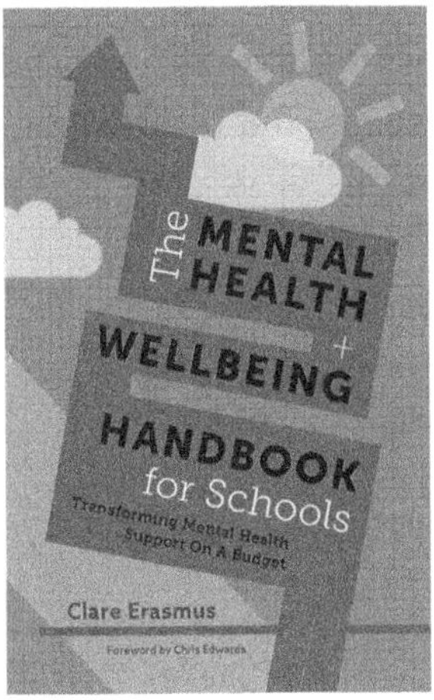

The Mental Health and Wellbeing Handbook for Schools

Transforming Mental Health Support on a Budget

Clare Erasmus

Foreword by Chris Edwards

Paperback: £16.99/$24.95
ISBN: 978 1 78592 481 1
eISBN: 978 1 78450 869 2
144 pages

This book lays out an intuitive and practical approach to mental health and wellbeing that any school can adopt to transform their mental health support for students.

With a focus on providing staff with practical tools on a limited budget, the book helps schools make a real difference to student mental health. It sets out a roadmap for staff to create robust mental health support for students without requiring qualifications in psychology or counselling. It covers key areas including staff training, creating safe spaces for wellbeing and how to harness the support of parents and the local community. It also includes practical advice for addressing concerns such as stress, self-harm and body image.

From small, everyday improvements that foster a culture of mental wellbeing to whole school campaigns, this book shows how to embed mental health at the heart of a school's philosophy.

Clare Erasmus has 20 years' teaching experience and is director of mental health and wellbeing at Brighton Hill Community School and creator of the TED talk #familyMH5aday. She currently lives in Portsmouth, UK.

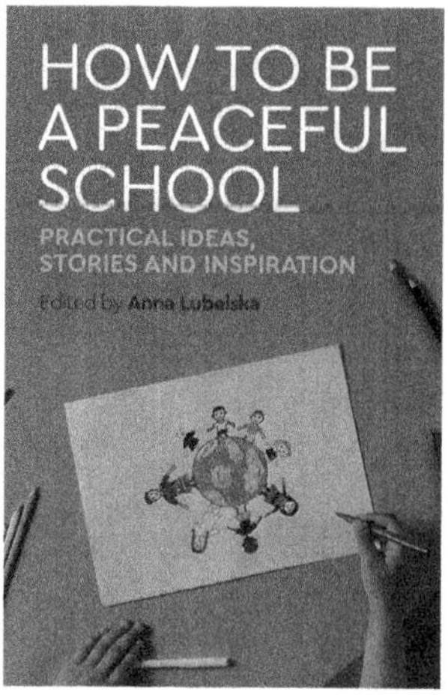

How to Be a Peaceful School

Practical Ideas, Stories and Inspiration

Edited by Anna Lubelska

Paperback: £14.99/$24.95
ISBN: 978 1 78592 156 8
eISBN: 978 1 78450 424 3
224 pages

Peace is needed now more than ever in schools, by pupils and teachers alike. This inspiring guide provides primary, secondary and special schools with practical methods to improve pupil and teacher wellbeing, combat bullying, and promote peace both inside and outside the school gates.

The founder of the Peaceful Schools Movement, Anna Lubelska, has brought together ideas and stories from teachers and charity workers to present a simple four step system for promoting positive peace in individuals, relationships, the school community and the world. It covers how to reduce stress, promote positive mental health, resolve conflict, nurture the potential of each individual, and encourage children to develop peacemaking skills and values. This holistic resource is equally beneficial for children and staff, and transforms school environments for the better.

Anna Lubelska is a passionate peace advocate. She is the founder of the Peaceful Schools Movement and of the charity Spiritual England, and former Head of Education at the Association for London Government.

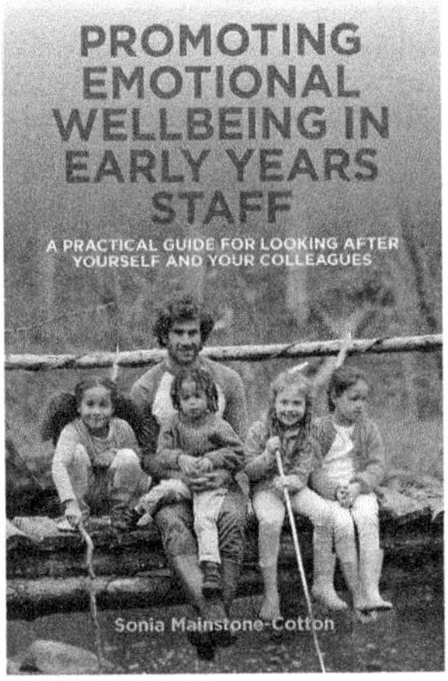

Promoting Emotional Wellbeing in Early Years Staff

A Practical Guide for Looking after Yourself and Your Colleagues

Sonia Mainstone-Cotton

Paperback: £14.99/$21.95
ISBN: 978 1 78592 335 7
eISBN: 978 1 78450 656 8
128 pages

Though children's wellbeing is high on the agenda for policy makers, the welfare of the professionals looking after them is often taken for granted. Sonia Mainstone-Cotton recognises that in order to enhance children's emotional wellbeing, it's vital that early years professionals are stress-free and emotionally well themselves. This is the first guide of its kind, offering succinct and practical guidance, tips and ideas for those working with young children on how to comfortably manage the pressures of their job, improve their work/life balance, and support the wellbeing of their colleagues. Easy to dip in and out of, this guide is an essential item for any early years staff room.

Sonia Mainstone-Cotton is a freelance trainer, consultant, nurture worker, and author of Promoting Young Children's Emotional Health and Wellbeing. She has worked with young children for over 25 years.

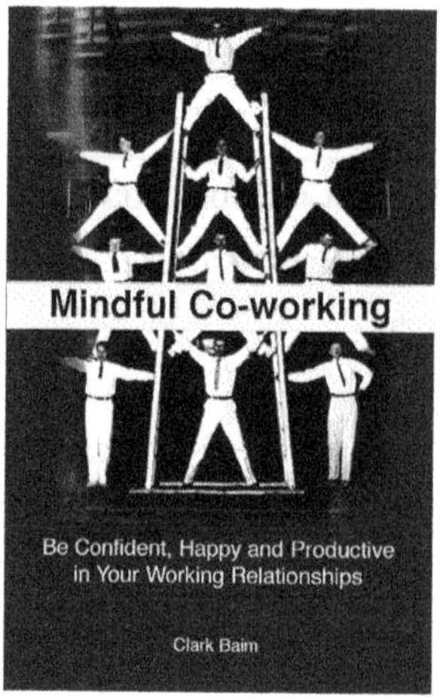

Mindful Co-Working

Be Confident, Happy and Productive in Your Working Relationships

Clark Baim

Paperback: £14.99/$24.95
ISBN: 978 1 84905 413 3
eISBN: 978 0 85700 803 9
176 pages

Transform and enhance your working relationships through mindful co-working.

Are you making the most of your co-working relationships?

Most of us work with others and spend as much time with colleagues as we do with our families - so it's important our working relationships run smoothly. By helping workers become more attuned to their colleagues, mindful co-working removes the pressure and stress of competition from working relationships to make them both more enjoyable and more effective. Author Clark Baim shares the secrets he has learned with co-workers and co-trainers during more than 2,000 training workshops. He also includes practical exercises and useful tools to help you perfect the art, whatever field you work in.

This indispensable guide to co-working is required reading for anyone who wants to work confidently with colleagues - and enjoy it!

Clark Baim has 25 years of experience working internationally as a trainer, group leader, supervisor and consultant working with organizational change. He is a registered psychotherapist and senior trainer with the British Psychodrama Association, and he is Co-Director of Change Point Ltd., which offers staff training in a wide variety of organizations. He is also Co-Director of the Birmingham Institute for Psychodrama. Clark has published extensively on supervision, groupwork methods, psychotherapy, attachment theory, applied theatre and offender treatment.